The Art of Self Acceptance

Powerful Methods for Overcoming Self-Doubt, Low Self-Esteem and Rejection

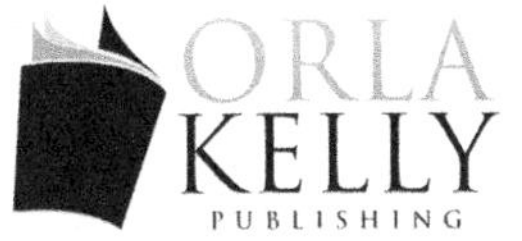

Gavin Meenan

978-1-914225-35-2

Published in Ireland by Orla Kelly Publishing.

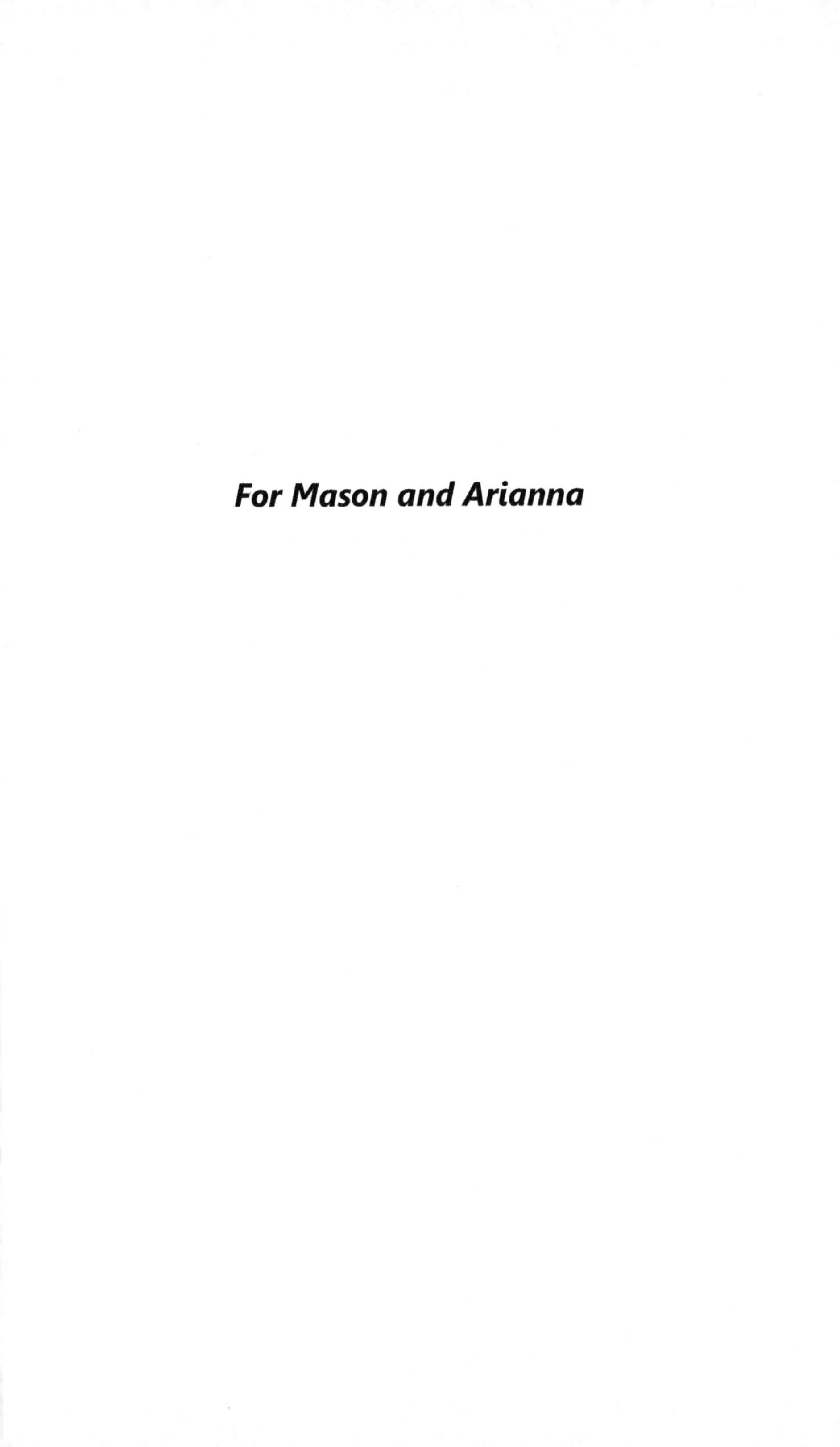

For Mason and Arianna

Contents

Introduction

Before We Begin

French philosopher Blaise Pascal once said the following:

> *"All of man's problems stem from his inability to sit quietly in a room alone".*

Hailed as one of the greatest thinkers of his time, this is as true today as it was back in the 1600s. In our hyper-distracted, hyper-productive, hyper-driven world, contentment is the enemy. You should never settle for what you are, who you are or what you have - you need more. Whether that's more money, more possessions, more relationships, more respect, more social standing or more entertainment, the story plays out the same. We never have enough. We never are enough.

And no matter what satisfaction we experience along the way, we anxiously await the arrival of the day when we'll achieve our goals and finally attain success (whatever that looks like to you).

But this isn't a book about minimalism. I'm not talking about "learning to settle" or "letting go of the material" so that you can begin to appreciate the riches of your inner world. That's not me - and I'm definitely **not** the man to write that kind of book.

If you're reading this, there's a good chance you already know who I am. I've been pretty open about my struggles in the past. In my life, I've battled with porn addiction, low self-esteem, substance dependency (not full-fledged alcoholism... let's call it "an unhealthy reliance"), raising a family, providing for them, finding meaning when I wasn't able to do so and more.

Your story may be different. For your own sake, I hope you've never experienced the same things I have. And the same is true for you - you've likely gone through specific trials in your life that I've never encountered. But I don't think that matters. While our struggles may differ in form, we're united by their impact.

Over the past 7 years, I've dived deep into figuring out what exactly has driven the various self-destructive and negative behaviours I've indulged in throughout my life:

- Crippling shyness as a child.
- Anxious nights where I lay awake and wondered if my parents would come home alive from a routine journey.
- Sexual frustration as a teenager (and the lies I told to compensate).
- My struggles with porn addiction.
- How dependent I grew on alcohol and the mask of confidence it gave me.
- How inadequate I thought I was, deep down.

- The way I used that pain as a catalyst for personal growth as I pursued - and attained - a European Powerlifting title.

- Trying to raise my children to be strong, healthy individuals when I felt I **barely** met that criteria myself.

- Providing for my family when I couldn't hold down a job.

- Struggling to find meaning as a stay-at-home dad.

- Believing I had nothing to offer other men as a coach.

As each new obstacle presented itself, I've engaged with it. I've striven to understand what drove those behaviours - what made me so unable to "sit quietly in a room alone".

And after a great deal of reflection, I've found an answer. One that's helped me to **finally** come to terms with who I am underneath... and one that's allowed me to turn the tide against these problems ever arising again.

This book is for anyone who

wants to enact real change in their lives. ☑

(like me) has struggled with addiction, low self-esteem

self-sabotages at every twist and turn. ☑

is ready to confront the reasons why self-improvement is so hard. ☑

Like I said, I'm no guru. I don't have the ultimate solution to all of life's problems. But what I do have is experience. It's up to you to decide if you can benefit from the lessons I've learned along the way.

Here's what I believe:

- You can't escape the problems caused by a weak foundation. Any character weaknesses you have will be exposed eventually. Whether the reckoning comes in the form of a difficult external situation or the mere passage of time, anything you build on unstable ground is going to crumble and fall. Guaranteed.

- You can't live the life you know you're capable of living until you face these problems head-on. Without doing so, you'll fall prey to the same self-destructive tendencies that you've always struggled with.

- **Rejection** (and the fear of it) creates the weak foundation that causes all your problems.

That last point might seem strange to you. But it's the most critical insight you could take from this book. So that's exactly where we'll start.

The Fear of Rejection (And Rejection Itself) Drives All You Do

On my journey of self-discovery, I've found that my inability to accept myself for who I am was the root cause of all my problems. Rather than face the hard truth that I was a flawed individual (but one who could change), I covered up my deficiencies.

Whether it was something that I had control over or not, I sought to hide it from the world. I over-compensated. I indulged in escapist behaviours - anything to get momentary relief from the painful situation I found myself in.

My personal turning point came when I realised that all along, rejection (and the fear of it) had been my Achilles heel.

I feared rejection by wider society, so I hid my perceived shortcomings. I struggled to fulfil the role of stoic provider my upbringing moulded me for. I did all the things that unspoken societal norms whispered I should.

I feared rejection by my peers (something anyone who was bullied as a child can relate to). So I covered up who I was. Starting from a young age, I built a facade to hide behind: an arrogant, brash, ladies' man who was the life of the party. I made up stories to paper over my lack of experience with women. Later, continuing into adulthood, I hid my true feelings from moment to moment, never wanting to expose who I really was.

I feared romantic rejection, so I tried to be the man I thought a good partner would want me to be. I never argued - rather than addressing conflict in the moment, I would swallow my words and instead let that resentment fester. And there was no question about "being myself". That guy wouldn't get the time of day, so he was pushed down, covered up with a mask of what I thought I should be. And, needless to say, my sexual frustration and the inadequacy I felt drove me towards porn (but we'll get into that, don't worry).

I rejected my thoughts and emotions. Anything I deemed inappropriate was repressed. I had been raised to believe that good people behaved in a certain way and judged those who didn't meet those criteria. For instance, they didn't get angry and they always put the needs of others above their own. I harnessed that pain to achieve an outward appearance of success... but failed to address the real problems underneath.

Finally, I rejected myself. Layer upon layer of external rejection (real, potential and perceived) disconnected me from who I really was. I took the judgements of others and turned them into *my* judgements. Rather than addressing the sense of purposelessness I felt, I ignored it. Rather than accepting those negative aspects of myself I couldn't change, I tried to cover them up. I overcompensated for those perceived shortcomings. Ditto for those things about myself that I could have changed if I truly cared. It was easier to slap a Band-Aid on the gaping wound than to amputate the limb altogether.

Some of the rejection I feared was real, rooted in actual experience. Some of it was perceived (i.e. I thought I had been rejected, but it may not have been the case whatsoever). But much of it was not rejection at all, merely the **fear** of it.

Even when the rejection was real, the question remains - so what? Why was that such a bad thing? The consequences of rejection (these days, at least) are fairly minimal. Looking back now, I would have traded all of the fake friendships, worthless days and drunken nights I had for the chance to be true to myself.

There's a book called "The Top 5 Regrets of the Dying", written by a woman called Bonnie Ware. As a palliative care nurse, her job was to attend to people who were terminally ill and living out their last few days on Earth. And in her book, she explains that the following five regrets cropped up again and again:

1. "I wish I'd had the courage to live a life true to myself, not the life that others expected of me"

2. "I wish I hadn't worked so hard"

3. "I wish I'd had the courage to express my feelings"

4. "I wish I had stayed in touch with my friends"

5. "I wish that I had let myself be happier"

Can you see how the fear of rejection is a key contributor to several of those regrets? And can you see why learning to overcome this fear is so important?

The truth is that, no one knows when their time will come. Hopefully, it's many years from now, when you've had the chance to live a rich, full life that brought you the happiness you're looking for. But whenever that time comes, I want you to be able to look back on a life well-lived... not to regret the fears that kept you shackled to a mediocre existence for so long.

By learning to overcome this fear of rejection, you'll be empowered. Maybe for the first time in years. You can read this book in a day, if you've got the time. But whether you devour it in one sitting or spread it out for as long as you need... when you truly make these paradigm shifts, you'll start to see benefits **immediately**.

You'll see it the very next morning, when you find yourself getting involved in that important conversation at work.

You know that you've got a lot to offer. And your fear of looking stupid in front of your "superiors"? *Nothing but a figment of your imagination*.

You'll see it a few weeks from now, when your friends start to notice how much more relaxed you are. They haven't said anything outright, but you notice them starting to treat you differently. And before long, they're coming to you for advice.

A few months after that, you see the impact of your newfound mindset on your paycheck. No longer fearful of putting yourself out there, you were confident enough to ask your boss for a raise. Given your recent improvements in performance, it was more than justified - and who knows? Maybe you'll put the extra money into a savings account so you can finally start your own business, like you've always wanted to.

At home, things are different too. Your partner, your kids, your extended family - they've all seen a new side to you. You're calmer. More confident. You're open with them and they know they can rely on you. You've never felt so at peace. Life hasn't become any less challenging, but you're in a much better position to deal with the everyday problems that arise.

Think of all the benefits you could experience in just a few short months... then expand the timeline. A year from now. 5 years from now. A decade. 50 years from now.

Living a good life - one you can look back on and be happy with - starts with overcoming that fear of rejection. Of accepting yourself for who you really are. Of becoming **unshakeable,** safe in the knowledge that you're enough.

With that in mind, let's look at what's in store.

How much is *really* there to say about rejection?

As it turns out, quite a bit. "Rejection" is an umbrella term for so many negative human experiences, it's almost impossible to accurately narrow it down. To that end, I've had to invent my own categories/styles of rejection just to make sense of it all. We'll be using those categories as a framework for approaching the topic.

In this framework, the four key categories of rejection are:

1. **Social Rejection:** rejection of identity as viewed through the eyes of society. ("*There is something wrong with the way I act.*")

2. **Romantic Rejection:** rejection of romantic/sexual identity as viewed through the eyes of others *or* rejection of the self as viewed through the eyes of a loved one. ("*There is something wrong with who/what I am.*")

3. **Personal Rejection:** a rejection of surface-level desires triggered by external judgements. ("*There's something wrong with my interests.*")

4. **Core Rejection:** a rejection of core desires/vision triggered by external judgements turned internal. ("*There's something wrong with my existence.*")

Very broad strokes, I know and some categories seem like they should be lumped in with others; but it'll make sense when we get to it, I swear!

To further break the issue of rejection down, I'm also going to run with the model that all rejection occurs because of two reasons:

1. *Societal reasoning* (i.e. when you're rejected because of who you are)

2. *Emotional reasoning* (i.e. when you're rejected because of something you've done)

This is an important distinction between rejection types, so make sure you understand the difference before proceeding.

Over the course of this book, I'll explain the worldviews that let me overcome my fear of rejection and ultimately allowed me to accept myself for who I was.

Through analysis of each rejection category, we'll be looking at:

- Why rejection is a fact of life.
- Why rejection hurts.
- How to stop letting the pain of rejection control you.

My goal isn't just to have you nod along and appreciate how smart I sound. It's to help you gain **your** unique insights.

My story might be different to yours, but I believe there are valuable lessons to be learned from the struggles of others. No matter your situation, pain is pain. By telling you what I've learned through my trials, you'll find something that will help you find your way too.

This is not going to be a highly scientific piece of work. I'm not going to speak down to you from my high horse, telling you why you're to blame for all your troubles and that I (being the perfect man I am) know exactly what you should do to stop suffering.

Again - I'm not that kind of man, and this is not that kind of book.

My aim is to write something highly usable. Something that will help you gain perspective you didn't have before. Something that will enable you to start **fixing** those foundational problems - before they can cause serious damage. Or, if they've already caused you real harm, then to help you move on and grow.

Most crucially, you'll learn the insights that helped me gain clarity: hard-won, but vital.

I encourage you to read this book through chapter by chapter. Doing so will help you to get a better sense of how conflict in your external world causes problems internally - and vice versa. I've deliberately kept each section brief to ensure that you get maximum return on your time. That said, if you think one section in particular could help you, feel free to jump right in.

What Lies Ahead

As an expansion to the brief explanation above, here's a high-level overview of the four-part journey you're about to go on:

1. **Social rejection**: In this section, we'll talk about the impact of your peer group (past and present) on your development. Rejection by your peers can have a long-lasting influence on you, particularly if it occurs when you're a child. Even as an adult, the desire to fit in with your friends can be hard to shake. By learning how the fear of social rejection holds you back, you'll be able to loosen its grip on your psyche once and for all.

2. **Romantic rejection**: In this section, we'll talk about how the fear of rejection in a romantic context shapes your behaviour. This is something I've had a lot of experience with, and I can tell you now - **nothing** fucks you up quite like feeling you'll never be "good enough" for your partner. By learning to combat rejection-based fear in this area, you'll set yourself up to live a much happier life.

3. **Personal rejection:** In this section, we're going to talk about what happens when you reject your surface-level thoughts and desires. Fearing the judgment of others, many of us suppress elements of ourselves that we think are less desirable. "Nerdy" or "girly" hobbies, unconventional styles of speech or dress... like robots, we accept the rejection programming of others and let it dictate everything about how we live. But rejecting so many surface-level desires only leads to repression and emotional damage. Learning how to engage with yourself, your wants and - most importantly - your *needs* is crucial to building a happy life.

4. **Core rejection**: In this section, we'll talk about how being out of touch with your core causes serious problems - the kind that show up in all other areas of your life. For instance, I've seen countless men struggle to find purpose in life. This commonly arises when they've failed to identify their mission (something significant they can dedicate themselves to). Because they don't understand **who they are** at a deep level - or worse, because

> they **reject** themselves at that deepest level - they struggle to make meaningful progress in any area of their lives. Whether they reject their core consciously or unconsciously, the damage this causes is substantial. When you act in alignment with your core self, life gets better. Taking the right actions is simpler, you're more productive and you feel happier on a day-to-day basis.

While my perspective is obviously rooted in personal experience, I'll also draw on the stories of others and outside research to support my points wherever needed. And at the end of each section, we'll bring it back to how you can use the information to improve **your** situation. Because that's all that truly matters - that you find something here that helps you live a better life.

So, without further ado, let's get started.

1
Social Rejection

What is Social Rejection?

It may sound like a redundant question at first - but with a term as vague as 'social rejection', it's important to clarify exactly what we're talking about. Ultimately, all rejections are 'social rejections'. Rejection, by nature, is a social act. But when I use the term 'social rejection' in this book, you can take it to mean '*rejection in social situations of a platonic nature.*'

For our purposes, the term will be used to refer to instances such as:

- A falling out with a friend
- Schoolyard bullying
- Workplace bullying

- Being snubbed from an invitation to a party
- Exclusionary behaviours/shunning by peers or colleagues
- Being demeaned, insulted or harassed by peers/ superiors in public

The reason we're using such a broad term for a (relatively) specific category is that the dynamics of platonic, romantic and internal rejection all differ greatly from one another, while the dynamics of the examples listed above are relatively similar. Being bullied and falling out with a friend are two very different situations - but the motivations behind each are often the same and usually occur in the same environments. Because of this, it makes sense to examine them together.

I'll be straight with you. *Societal norms* are the most common root of social rejection. Most bullying, harassment and exclusionary behaviour on a platonic level occur due to preconceived beliefs we're taught during childhood - a dislike for the different, so to speak. It's rare that children bully each other as a consequence of hurt feelings or offense - more often than not, children and adults are bullied because they are "othered" by their peers. The logic of this "othering" is rooted almost solely in societal norms.

Humans are social animals. In the past, we formed tribes of hunters and gatherers, building forts and strongholds to protect ourselves from other tribes and the dangers of the natural world. Because resources like food and water are fundamentally limited, different tribes generally did not accept each other - to do so would have been to threaten their own status. Even if it would have made more sense to come together and form a *larger* settlement or stronghold, most tribes would choose to stay weak over having to come to terms with a group so 'different' from them.

"Othering" in modern times occurs due to this misguided survival instinct. In the past, "others" posed a genuine threat to survival. Other tribes might kill you, steal your food or destroy your homes. Because of this, surrounding yourself with people who were the same as you became extremely important.

“We know they’re not like us because they don’t ______ like we do. They’re our enemies.”

“We know you are like us because you ______ like we do. You’re our friend.”

As society evolved over the next several thousand years, the threat ‘others’ posed to our survival became much less significant - but that instinct to form communities of sameness didn’t.

Without isolated forts and leaders to rally behind, humans began to live in accordance with their wealth, profession or religion. We still see this in good/bad neighbourhoods nowadays. We began to dress in a certain way so that our ‘tribe’ could be identified, as with the ‘noble colours’ of the Middle Ages and branded clothes of the here and now. Symbols of social status (expensive clothes, cars, and jewellery) are our tribe identifiers nowadays, and their absence is often used as an excuse for social rejection.

That’s why children are bullied for dressing wrong or sounding stupid; because they’re viewed as being *fundamentally different* to the bully, they're not part of the same tribe. That makes them an appropriate target for aggression.

It's a bold claim to make, but I'm making it anyway: *nearly every platonic social rejection can be traced back to tribalism.* The reason for this is that before you've ever even *spoken* to a person, they've made a bunch of assumptions about you that colour how you'll be perceived. They're shallow assumptions (literally only skin-deep!) but have a profound impact on how that person will think of you going forward.

If you look roughly to be in the same tribe as them, they'll be much more open to you than if their gut instinct names you an 'other'. Factors which may contribute to this judgement include:

- Your skin colour
- Your general appearance (tattoos, piercings, hair colour)
- Your religion or lack thereof

- Your gender
- Your financial status
- Your accent/fluency in their language
- Your body language or posture

For the record, I think this judgement is totally unfair - but it'd be naive to say it doesn't happen. Hopefully, this'll change. As time passes and the world becomes more globalised, the number of people who'll have strong gut reactions to skin colours, accents or sexualities will naturally decrease. Maybe they won't be used as excuses to discriminate in the future. But even if all the factors listed above vanish, we'll still be pre-emptively judging each other - just for hobbies or shoe size, instead.

It's human instinct to judge others. We all do it, whether or not we're aware of it. That instinct kept us safe for millennia when times weren't so safe. But in the modern world, preconceived judgements are unhelpful more often than not and actively detrimental when they cloud our judgement of a person.

Shaped By Shoulds - The Rules (Spoken and Unspoken) That Define Us

By the time you take your first steps, say your first words or get into your first toddler fist-fight over who *really* owns that fire truck, your behaviour has already been informed and influenced by society. As you grow up, this doesn't change much. You learn that:

- You should listen to authority figures
- You should stay quiet unless spoken to or called on
- You should do your homework
- You should play sports, play an instrument and play nice with others
- You should eat everything on your plate
- You should be grateful for everything you have
- You should do **this**, not **that**

And so on. Lots of Shoulds, but very little explanation for **why** value has been ascribed to certain things and not others.

As you grow into a teenager, you might start to rebel against the Shoulds imposed upon you from a young age. But even this rebellion takes place along well-defined contrarian lines:

- You **should** drink, smoke or take other substances
- You **should** do things your parents think you shouldn't do
- You **should** dress in line with the people you want to fit in with
- You **should** always strive to impress others
- You **should** start pursuing romantic partners - the more, the more adventurous, the better
- You **shouldn't** focus on performing well in school - who cares!
- You **should** focus on performing well in school - it's your future!

In seeking to break free from the chains that bind you, you end up swapping one set of Shoulds for another.

And as you grow older still, an entirely different set of Shoulds come to the fore:

- You **should** go to college and study something "worthwhile" (e.g. engineering, business, science)
- You **should** get a good job after you graduate
- You **should** work 40 hours a week until you retire
- You **should** settle down, find someone to marry and raise a family
- You **should** be happy - lots of people have it worse than you
- You **should** raise your kids to fit into the system, just like you were raised

Obviously, the journey above is greatly simplified. And it's not as if you wake up one day, are handed a list of these rules and are trapped by them for the rest of your life. The reality is far more insidious than that. You only come to these realisations gradually, if at all.

Another point to note is that all of the Shoulds listed above are common examples of **societal norms**. Some are explicit, easily recognised - others are far more difficult to discern.

Awareness is the First Step

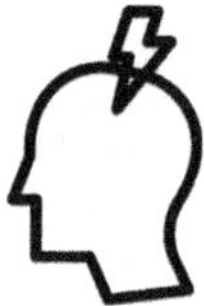

We all live in accordance with a list of Shoulds. These rules (spoken or unspoken) guide our thoughts, behaviours and ultimately... our **results.** The life we're living right now can be attributed to the rules we live by.

Even if it's possible to do so, I don't think there's any benefit in living totally free of rules. Without effective guiding principles, how can you make good decisions? How can you ensure that you stay on the path towards achieving your goals?

The answer to both of these questions is the same - you **can't**. We need those rules to create the life we want to live. But unless you're intelligently choosing those rules for yourself, you will consistently bump up against invisible roadblocks.

Before you can remove these obstacles from your life and break free of the Shoulds that bind you, you need to be **aware** of them. And, in my experience, awareness often starts with solitude.

Solitude takes many forms. It's likely you're already engaging in some practice that affords you solitude. If you've ever:

- Taken a drive down familiar roads to clear your head
- Gone to the gym to take your mind off things
- Laid down in the middle of the day to take a quick break

- Spent too long in the shower because you were lost in thought

Then you know what I'm talking about.

People meditate, write in journals and engage in other mindful activities for exactly this purpose. They seek solitude - not just in the physical sense, but in the emotional and mental sense too. When you go for a long, ambling walk all by yourself, it's nice to just be in silence with your own thoughts. Maybe you like the sensation of being away from crowds. But I've always found that getting that **cognitive** breathing room is the real goal.

When you're bogged down in your day-to-day, it can be hard to see the bigger picture and make good decisions. Ryan Holiday's excellent book "Stillness is The Key" makes this very argument - solitude helps you think more clearly. That solitude doesn't have to be eternal and it doesn't have to be literal... but a sense of inner peace is an invaluable asset for attaining happiness, success and clarity of mind. With it, you're in a much better position to uncover the Shoulds that have a stranglehold on your psyche.

In the following sections of this book, you'll notice that I continually advocate for things like journalling, meditating and introspective walking. That's because:

1. I've personally benefited from these methods

2. Solitude is the best weapon you possess in the fight to break free of your fear of rejection **for good**

Writing has long been held as one of the best ways to clarify your thoughts on something. Personally, I find that overwhelming problems built up in my head become a lot more manageable when they're down on paper. Meditation is a classic - when you can bring your attention to focus on the breath and **nothing but the breath**, you're well on your way. And something about the physical, repetitive motion of low-impact exercise seems to unlock deeper insights then you'd get otherwise.

The form your solitude takes doesn't matter too much. If you've already got something that works for you, that's great! Keep putting it into practice and sharpen its edge with some of the tools you'll acquire throughout this book. And if you're looking for methods that suit you, then give journalling, meditating and walking a try.

Exercise

Uncover Your Shoulds by Asking Questions

Awareness is key. But unless you take some time to reflect upon what your rules may be, you can't hope to uncover them.

The act of regularly assessing your guiding principles can come in the form of conversations with a trusted friend or mentor. It could be an internal conversation you have as you take a long, ambling walk by yourself. It could be a regular 30 minutes of journalling last thing at night, as you process the events of the day. It could even be a quiet 5 minutes of reflection first thing in the morning, before the chaos of everyday life snatches your attention away.

Regardless of the form it takes, regular examination of your rules is vital. Without engaging in this practice, you won't be able to eliminate those roadblocks that prevent you from making progress.

For instance, here are 25 simple questions you can use to get the ball rolling. I've personally found questions exactly like these to be helpful in determining what my rules are (even when I couldn't consciously vocalise them). Write them, say them out loud, have a friend pose them to you - do whatever you need to do to get your answers.

Your Perspective on Wealth and Money

1. Do you believe "your wealth is your health"?

2. Do you believe "it takes money to make money"?

3. Do you think it's possible for someone to get rich in an ethical manner?

4. Are all millionaires exploitative? How about billionaires?

5. Are you happy with how much money you make? Why/why not?

Your Perspective on Risk

1. Do you believe that taking risks is important?

2. Do you believe that it's "better to be safe than sorry"?

3. Do you think that it's "better to have loved and lost than to have never loved at all?"

4. Do you think it's dangerous to "put all your eggs in one basket"?

5. Do you think "double or nothing" is a good strategy?

Your Perspective on Religion and Morality

1. Do you have any religious faith?

2. Do you feel it's important to have religious faith?

3. Do you think that some actions and behaviours make a person more "worthy" than others?

4. Do you believe "what goes around, comes around"?

5. Do you believe that morality is relative? Or absolute?

Your Perspective on Romance/Sexuality

1. Do you believe that you need to get married?

2. What do you think of lifelong bachelors?

3. Do you think it's important that you have lots of sexual partners?

4. Do you think it's important that your partner **hasn't** had lots of sexual partners?

5. Do you think men and women are equal?

Your Perspective on Family

1. Do you feel it's important to stay close to your family?

2. Do you respect your parents?

3. Do you love your family?

4. Do you feel it's important to have kids of your own?

5. Do you think it's possible to be truly happy with or without a family?

These questions aren't complicated. In fact, you might read some of them and roll your eyes. But the answers you provide to them can be illuminating. They provide an insight into the deep-rooted beliefs you hold in various areas of your life... the kind of things you seldom consider, if ever.

Think of these questions as a starting point to understanding and recontextualising social rejection. The trick is learning that *social rejection is almost always not about you.* It's about *society*. The reason you were rejected as a kid for liking the wrong soccer team wasn't that there was something wrong with your choice - it's just tribalism. The rejecter feared connection with someone different to them and didn't have the tools to dismantle their own immature judgement. You weren't denied an invitation to that wedding because you're a bad person, but because you were viewed as *different* somehow to the category of people the couple wished to invite.

In both of these cases, the rejection *is not your fault.*

That doesn't mean it's not painful - but the reason it hurts comes from the same place the rejection does: *the human need to belong*. Learning to dismantle that social structure and untangle your sense of personal culpability is the key to healing social rejection. The only social rejection you're at 'fault' for - and that's unhelpful language to begin with - is one you've caused through cruelty or callousness. The blame for all others lies with the rejecters themselves.

An Example of Social Rejection

Take a class of 20 ten-year old students. Each has a unique mix of abilities and attributes; some are academic and quiet, others are confident and excitable. They all have their own circle of friends they play with, both in and out of school and get on well together as a group.

Say you're one of these students. You're outgoing, bright and chatty. You're friends with everyone, even the ones who disliked you when you were younger. You don't hold a grudge against anyone for anything, and you're well-liked by all your teachers.

But one day, invitations to George's birthday party are handed out and you don't get one. You can't understand why. You play soccer with George every day at school - you've been to George's house and George has been to yours. You support the same team, you have the same friends and you're thinking of going

> to the same secondary school. So why have you been passed over?
>
> You ask George why this has happened. George, understandably, is uncomfortable and won't give a straight answer. This greatly upsets you. When you go home, you tell your mother what's happened and ask her to talk to George's mother for you. When she does, George's mother gives an explanation for the rejection - "*we thought your son would feel bad if he saw everyone else giving more expensive presents than him.*"

In this scenario, the rejection is not ultimately malicious. However, it was both:

A. Outside the rejected person's control (As a ten-year old you cannot control either your family's social status *or* how people perceive it)

B. Entirely disconnected from the behaviour and personality of the rejected person (your friendliness, charm and politeness were not at fault - it was a matter of how your family is perceived)

And despite the fact that it wasn't malicious, you're still hurt by it. From this scenario, you learn for the first time that your wealth/status are a barrier to the relationships you can form, and you internalise that you are worth less than your classmates because you are poorer than them. In the future, you go on to work a high-paying job to ensure this won't happen again - but money worries haunt you no matter where you go, and you're afraid not to spend it on partners in case they abandon you.

You've internalised this rejection. And unless you take counteraction, you'll be saddled with this burden for the rest of your life.

How Social Rejection is Internalised

The reason social rejection is damaging is not the consequences of the rejection itself, but how it's interpreted by the rejected party. Humans have a need for a certain amount of socialisation, sure, but that doesn't mean we biologically *need* a crowd's acceptance to be happy. If you work with 15 people and only 5 of them like you, you could still have a perfectly fulfilling social life... hell, you'd be fine with just 1!

So why does social rejection hurt so much?

Simply put, social rejection hurts because of what we learn from it. If your friendship is rejected because you're the wrong height (for some bizarre reason), you'll internalise the event as proof that *"I am not tall enough."* In the example above, you internalised your lack of a party invitation as proof that you weren't *"rich enough to make real friends,"* and later that you weren't *"worthy enough to make real friends."* The fact that no one told you the whole office was going for drinks after work doesn't hurt because they're your only potential friends in the whole world. It hurts because you internalise their judgement as your own. It goes a little like this:

"They don't want me around unless I have to be" → "They don't like me" → "I am not someone who deserves to be liked" → "I don't like myself."

Here's where your subconscious kicks in... and things get tricky. It doesn't just control our thoughts - it controls what thoughts we can and can't have. It's the foundation of our consciousness. And when we're rejected by someone, our subconscious repeats the rejection over and over in our own mind's voice until the message has been internalised and incorporated into our personality.

Have you ever lain awake at night thinking about an awkward situation you can't forget? You can thank your subconscious for that. It takes the raw data of a rejection, converts it to a personal value judgement and plays it on loop until you accept it and make an appropriate change to your behaviour.

The key to healing social rejection lies in breaking that loop - which I'll delve into more later. But as a quick spoiler for you all, the answer is two words I'm sure you're sick of hearing:

Introspection *and* mindfulness

Or, in other words, you'll have to do a lot more stuff like the exercise above.

2
Romantic Rejection

What is Romantic Rejection?

What a question that is - and one I'm pretty sure everybody's got an answer to, ranging from "painful, but part of life" to "something I encounter every Saturday night".

To massively oversimplify it, let's say there are two main types of romantic rejection. The first is rejection that comes when trying to *establish* a romantic bond - i.e. you approach someone in a nightclub and get shot down. The second type is rejection that comes during a romantic relationship - at its most extreme, this might be a breakup or divorce.

If it helps, you can call the first *anticipatory rejection* and the second, *reactionary rejection*.

But whatever label and logic you put on it, it's hard to overstate how damaging romantic rejection can be. It can be a massive blow to confidence and self-esteem. It can also very quickly become a cycle - somebody who's just been shot down in a club will make their next approach less confidently, almost anticipating the rejection this time and are more likely to get it because they're carrying themselves worse. There's a reason some people get into bad relationships over and over again. It's not just being unlucky in love - it's that the initial romantic rejections they suffered gave them an unsteady foundation to build a relationship on in the first place. Without fixing that foundation, they'll keep making the same mistakes.

Basically, the confidence hit that comes from being rejected even *once* can have knock-on effects if you're not equipped to cope with it. Those knock-on effects will make it more likely for you to be rejected again if not taken care of and so on... which explains why rejections tend to come in a pattern. But why would somebody who ticks all the boxes be romantically rejected in the first place?

Anticipatory Romantic Rejection

Definition: *Rejection that occurs outside of a romantic relationship.*

To go back to our earlier example, let's explain the roots behind anticipatory romantic rejection. You approach someone in a nightclub. You have a conversation with them. You try to escalate things and you're rejected.

A common occurrence. But a mysterious one. Where *did* you go wrong?

There are a number of places. Naturally, if your conversation is boring or if you don't distinguish yourself from other people, it's more likely you'll be rejected. But this isn't a book about how to 'game' the system, or what six alpha phrases to use to get one-night stands. So let's assume that every controllable factor about the approach - timing, conversation, etc. - was fine. What leads to rejection in *those* instances?

More often than not, anticipatory romantic rejection stems from societal norms, while reactionary romantic rejection stems from emotional reasoning. It's unlikely that the person you're approaching in the nightclub has been *hurt* by you doing so. In fact, most people will be flattered to receive honest attention, so long as you haven't made them uncomfortable beforehand. But flattered or not, the approached party often still rejects the approacher. The societal norms that may lead to this include:

- Shallow judgements of your appearance, including any based on race or ethnicity

- Judgements of your wealth, including those based on your clothing, skin, haircut, etc.

- Manners, mannerisms and countenance

- Body language and posture

Obviously, the most common reason for the rejection of an approach is that the person you're approaching isn't attracted to you. But attraction itself is shaped by nothing *but* societal norms - it's a pseudo-requirement for men to be tall and women to be slim due to standards pushed by the media and society at large. Some people will find different races unattractive by default, because of the historical idea that it's "improper" to mix outside your race. It doesn't matter if an individual agrees with this sentiment - growing up around people who do, can embed it in even the fairest person's subconscious.

Rejection based on attraction is a tricky topic to discuss. At the end of the day, it's a person's right to reject somebody they're not attracted to, wherever the reasons for that lack of attraction come from. But understanding why/how they're coming to that conclusion of no attraction can help to take the sting out of it, so it's still worth discussing.

As a personal trainer, I've worked with a lot of men who exercise just to make themselves more attractive. And there's nothing wrong with that. Really! It's good to know what you want and why. All the same, it's still sad to work with people who have a lot more going for them than they allow themselves to realise. Men who are 5'5 but in excellent shape; men who are in average shape but are extremely well-spoken; men with no hair but incredible confidence... the list goes on.

It's not unfair for anyone to reject someone based on attractiveness - the act itself isn't *morally wrong.* But that doesn't change the hurt the rejected party might feel, and it's alright for them to feel a little cheated or bitter about it.

It's no one's fault that society puts tall men and slim women on a pedestal... but it's still crap that shorter men and bigger women have to deal with the baggage.

Romantic rejections based on appearance (most anticipatory rejections, basically, since all they've got to judge you by is appearance) always sting, whether it's for a feature that's in your control or not. But as with social rejection, the damage comes when the rejection is internalised as an unshakeable truth. It goes from:

"She's rejected me because I'm unattractive." → "I'm unattractive." → "I'm unattractive to everyone." → "I'm not worthy of love."

But that conclusion isn't a reasonable one.

Ultimately, attractiveness is subjective. Any one person's opinion on it should be taken with a grain of salt - but so should the *crowd's* opinion.

As a social species, we find attractive what we're *told* to find attractive. To use a dramatic term, we're effectively brainwashed from a young age into understanding "beauty" as a set of very specific features. But these markers of attractiveness - high cheekbones, thick hair, well-defined muscles, large breasts - didn't come from anywhere sensible. They're just stories that people agree make sense for the moment.

I mean, look at King Henry VIII! Sure, he was a king, but he was also massively overweight and still had *six wives.* He's not alone in that. In the medieval era, being overweight was considered attractive because it proved you were wealthy enough to be well-fed. At the time, being skinny/lean was seen as *un*attractive (peasants were the first to go hungry). That's flipped around nowadays - which just goes to prove our point. Less than a thousand years have passed and what we deem attractive has entirely reversed.

(For a more contemporary example, think of how different the curvier body shape praised in the 1920s was vs. the stick-thin supermodel ideal of the 2000s. Total opposites, right?)

I'm sure there are people who'll disagree with me when I say this, but... I'd be inclined to say *"fuck it*" when it comes to worrying about how conventionally attractive you are. Is it harder to find a relationship if you don't meet societal ideals? Yeah. And does rejection for that reason still hurt? Of course. But you can't change your skin colour, accent or the body you've been born with.

All you can do is stay healthy, be the best you can be and strive to take it all on the (possibly too-small) chin.

It's their loss if they reject you because "your nose is huge". Not yours.

Reactionary Romantic Rejection

Definition: *Rejection that occurs once you're already in a relationship, i.e. a breakup*

In contrast to anticipatory romantic rejection, which is mostly based on societal ideals, break-ups are usually born from emotional reasoning.

I think it's fair to say that most break-ups occur due to one party being hurt by the other and/or losing interest in them. The reason I'm writing off societal factors as a significant contributor is that, by the time both parties have entered into a proper relationship, they'll be past most societal reasons for rejection. They'll already have mostly deemed each other suitable based on the external stuff like appearance, wealth, etc. Sure, these things can simmer under the surface and eventually boil over. That said, most breakups occur due to behaviour/action.

That, among other obvious reasons, is why being dumped hurts worse than having a one-night stand reject you.

You can use the reasons listed in the section above to re-contextualise a rejection in a nightclub. It's easy to understand how the rejected party is blameless for it. Through gaining this understanding, it's also possible to come to peace with the idea that you *will* be rejected, and that the rejection is no reason you shouldn't try again with someone else. But being broken up with on the basis of your behaviour, on who you actually *are*? That hurts. Especially if you actually agree with the reasoning.

But, as with the other kind of romantic rejection, there are two angles to take here. Either:

A. Your partner's reasoning is unfair or misguided.

They dump you over something that didn't happen/wasn't your true intention; it happened because they were bored, because they found someone new... in any of these cases, where the breakup truly wasn't because of something you did, that break-up says a lot more about your partner than you. If you've done nothing wrong and your partner still breaks up with you, the fault for that decision lies with them. Disentangling the guilt you feel will help you to see that and move on.

B. Your partner's reasoning is fair and accurate.

They're breaking up with you because you *have* wronged them, you *were* a bad partner and you both know it. In these cases, it's easy to wallow in self-pity - but you have to fight the temptation. Anyone who breaks up with you for these reasons has done you a huge favour. They've exposed a character flaw you may not have not seen otherwise and that gives you a chance to fix it.

You can strive to work on yourself while you heal, and become a better partner for the next person you enter into a relationship with. You can become more honest, more dedicated, more giving... while it hurts to have your issues spelled out by someone you love, you should take it as an opportunity for growth. The reason this kind of rejection hurts, more than anything else, is that it implies your partner has no faith that you won't make the same mistake again. This is especially true in cases where they leave right after revealing all these "obvious" character flaws. But they haven't done that to hurt you. They've done it because that's what's best for *them*. You need to respect that going forward. All you can do is strive not to let it happen again by correcting the issues that led to the breakup in the first place.

It's not as pretty a message as the previous one. It's less "*love yourself*" and more "*accept that things need to change*". But why can't the two go hand-in-hand? You can love yourself *while* you strive to improve; or better yet, strive to improve *because* you love yourself. If you know, deep down, that your behaviour led to the collapse of your relationship, then you also know what needs to change.

All that's left is to change it.

But I'm getting side-tracked - coaching you through a breakup isn't the point of this book. Remember: we're here to look at how the types of rejections impact more than surface level emotions, and how even the breakup of a two-week relationship can impact your psychological development.

How Romantic Rejection is Internalised

I'm sure that, by now, you're starting to understand how the subconscious takes rejection. It turns an exterior message ("You are _____") and transforms it to what *sounds like* internal truth ("I will always be ______.")

The problem with this system is that your subconscious is a dumbass. It takes the worst-case scenario and forces your acceptance of it to protect you from harm; both for self-preservation and preservation of the tribe, as discussed in the previous chapter.

Anticipatory romantic rejection is usually internalised as toxic self-talk. Having your offer of a date or exchange of numbers rejected is taken as proof of your unattractiveness and therefore as proof that you'll never find love. It goes a little like:

"No, I don't want to go on a date with you. Sorry." → *"I've been rejected because I'm ugly."* → "I'm ugly." → *"Nobody will ever love me because I'm ugly."* → *"I'm not worthy of love."* → *"I don't love myself."*

Reactionary rejection, on the other hand, has more direct effects on your behaviour when interpreted negatively. Toxic self-talk is still a huge element of this, but it's often also internalised through antisocial tendencies and emotional repression. It goes from:

"I'm breaking up with you because you lied to me." → *"I've been rejected because she's hurt by my dishonesty."* → *"My dishonesty hurt her."* → *"I'm a dishonest piece of shit."* → *"I don't deserve to find love."* → *"I don't love myself."*

Both types have the same endpoint, but different ways of getting there.

As with social rejection, it's *crucial* to remember that rejection is an active choice *somebody else takes.* It's something that happens *to* you as much as it does *because of* you. Many rejections are nobody's fault - they're a natural conclusion to a relationship that never really worked in the first place.

It's easy to internalise someone dumping you as proof that you're a piece of shit. It's even easier when they call you one. But even *if* they're right in their judgement of you, what use is there in accepting and resigning yourself to it? Strive to get so much better that nobody can ever rightly call you a piece of shit again. *Take it as a chance to grow.*

Work on yourself. Work on the problems that gave your relationship a rocky foundation to start with. Take the rejection as a learning opportunity... and move on.

Next time will be better

(Oh, and if you were wondering how you actually *do* the moving on? Well, I'm getting to that. But as another spoiler... it'll also involve *introspection* and *time.* Sorry if you were hoping for something quicker.)

3
Personal Rejection

What is Personal Rejection?

Personal Rejection, as a category, is the first form of "internal" rejection we've looked at so far. While the social and romantic rejection are external. They only take root when we internalise them. In contrast, personal rejection is internal by definition.

For our purposes, we can define personal rejection as the rejection of elements of our personality/our interests because of external pressure.

Personal Rejection is the result, when you tell a three-year old boy he's "wrong" to want to be a ballerina, or when ten-year olds tell each other it's "gay" to do XYZ. Being demeaned or pressured by others, leads a person to suppress vital elements of their interests or personality for the sake of fitting in. This leads to dissatisfaction, confusion and a general feeling of being inauthentic - because ultimately, that's what they *are* being.

As you've probably noticed from the description above, Personal Rejection sounds a *lot* like Social Rejection. And there's a good reason for that. Personal Rejection is another way of describing Social Rejection at its most severe. It's what happens when we accept the shallow external judgements of others as native truth.

As discussed earlier, Social Rejection comes about as a result of societal expectations being pushed onto others. The internalisation of these expectations triggers Personal Rejection. It goes like:

"*You don't act like us. We won't be friends with you!*" →
"*They won't be friends with me because I'm different.*" →
"*They won't be friends with me because of who I am.*" →
"*I need to change who I am if I want to have friends.*"

As with all rejection, your mileage may vary on this one. But while mentally strong individuals won't internalise Social Rejection so intensely, it'd be naïve to think that this only happens to a minority. Many children and adults suppress their true interests and personality for the sake of fitting in. We all know someone who does this: they're the people who hide their hobbies and talents to avoid ridicule, but pay the price by never getting to be themselves.

You probably don't need me to spell out why this is a bad thing. But if you do, just let me make one thing clear: *no matter* who you are, *no matter* how different you might be to society's ideal, you will *never* find true happiness unless you embrace yourself fully. Happiness cannot co-exist with self-rejection. If you ever want to find inner peace, it's crucial you learn to accept yourself for who you are - even if that's someone others have rejected in the past.

Obviously, I'm not talking about embracing cruelty or nasty thoughts here. But as long as being true to yourself doesn't cause harm to others, you need to embrace whoever that is as totally as you can.

This is probably a controversial topic, but as a parent, I feel very strongly about this issue. I've always believed that my children should be allowed to engage with any interest they choose. I never stop them experimenting with a hobby, fashion or pastime just so they fit the societal expectations of their gender, as I've seen so many other parents do. I'm not here to pass divine judgement on anybody else; to me, that kind of repression only leads to problems down the road.

But I care about this issue as more than just a parent. As a personal trainer, I've seen many clients fail to commit themselves fully to working on their bodies because they're afraid they'll be ridiculed for making the effort. In many cases, it's easier to stay as you are than to make a change, even if that means staying unhealthy. Passion, it seems, has gone out of vogue. It's cool not to care now.

And people are so afraid of having their identity questioned (or in other words, their place in the tribe questioned) that they deprive themselves of what they need to be - physically, emotionally and psychologically healthy.

Again... I'm sure I don't need to tell you why this is a problem.

What Does Personal Rejection Look Like?

Let's take a fairly basic example of Personal Rejection as a case study - one I'm sure many of you will be familiar with.

Pretending to watch Game of Thrones.

It sounds stupid, sure, but I couldn't tell you how many people I've had inform me in hushed tones that they've never seen a single episode, that they only pretended to watch the show so they wouldn't be interrogated by friends and colleagues.

Game of Thrones became such a cultural phenomenon in the last few years that it was nearly a sin to admit you'd never seen it. The decision to lie about having done so spread quicker than the show itself!

The same can be seen in people who pretend to watch sports, like certain kinds of music or who dress just to copy the people around them... We've all done this once or twice in our adult lives, though it seems like a school-yard thing at first blush. But what makes us do it?

Just like Social Rejection, it's all to do with fear. Fear of losing our place in the tribe, of being branded an "other". It's the primal anxiety of being cast out in the cold, although the chances of that happening in the modern world are a million to one. We're so terrified of being seen as anything other than completely run-of-the-mill, that we'll do anything to convince others we're like them.

We know it's not rational. In the 21st-century, it's not like being thrown out of the tribe means being torn apart by sabre-toothed tigers. But that safety doesn't change the risk of being socially isolated due to our differences. There are a *lot* of people out there who genuinely *avoid* being friends with anybody different to them.

But that's not a good argument for trying to fit in.

Although close-minded attitudes might be common, that doesn't mean they're *right.* Anybody who would end a friendship over a difference in interests isn't worthy of your time in the first place. I'm friends with a very diverse group of people, in terms of upbringing, interests, levels of fitness, worldviews... you name it, I've seen it.

And honestly, I think it's better this way - not having a shallow, surface-level commonality to bond over means that my friends *have* to be people I connect with on a deeper level. If I was only friends with somebody because we supported the same soccer club, I'm not sure I'd consider them much of a friend. There needs to be more to a relationship than having a few things in common - so if one of yours ends just because you *don't*, it probably wasn't one worth worrying about.

Again, this isn't about being contrarian for the sake of it. I'm not telling you to *inform* everybody you hate something they like. It's about not lying that you do. You can make conversation about things that don't interest you without having to resort to dishonesty. And besides, isn't it way more of a risk to be caught out for having lied to them? Even though you've done it to seem likeable, literally *nobody* wants to be friends with someone who does that. That's why you need to be honest about what you do and don't like.

Don't let the judgement of others prevent you from engaging with your truest self. If you want to behave in a way deemed either too-appropriate or too-inappropriate for your gender, forget the ones doing the deeming and *just do it*. Who cares if people think you're manly enough? That's just their perception and it's based on societal ideas that are as fictitious as boy/girl colours are.

There's no right or wrong way to be a man, and there's no right or wrong way to be a person. There's only authenticity and inauthenticity. Honesty and dishonesty. Strive to be authentic, strive to be honest and don't worry about the rest.

Anybody who doesn't accept you on those bases isn't worth your time in the first place.

How Personal Rejection is Internalised

Since Personal Rejection is internal by definition, it's extremely damaging when turned even further inwards. Where the internalisation of Social or Romantic Rejection (two forms of external rejection) leads to Personal Rejection, the further internalisation of Personal Rejection tells your subconscious that *you must not be who you really are.*

It's repression of the worst kind. Rejection of your fundamental self. It can start as early as childhood, where an education system forces us all into the same mould of academia and social engagement. It's further reinforced through media messages, bullying and peer pressure in adolescence, none of which go away in adulthood. We swap our school cliques for workplace cliques, swap the pressure of teachers for the pressure of bosses and end up living our whole lives in the shape others have chosen for us.

Since Personal Rejection of this kind can't occur without an external rejection to trigger it, the internalisation of personal rejection usually goes like this:

"We're rejecting you because you're different from us." (**SOCIAL REJECTION**.) → *"I've been rejected because I'm different from them."* → *"It's bad to be different from others."* → *"I should be the same as others."* (**PERSONAL REJECTION**.) → *"I need to change who I am."*

There's a reason that so many little boys and little girls tend to have the same interests as the rest of their gender, and I'm not talking about biology. It's because of societal pressures.

I've seen it myself many times. Parents stopping their children from buying the "wrong–gendered" toys in a shop, with a comment along the lines of "little boys/girls don't play with that, they play with *this*." The most recent example of this that I can remember is from around the time of the last *Avengers* release, in a Smyths Toys somewhere. I saw a mother telling her five-year-old daughter that she wasn't allowed to buy a figure of Iron Man because "that toy is only for boys." Naturally, the child didn't like this, started to cry and got bribed into silence by a Princess Fun Pak or something like that.

It's an innocuous enough situation, sure – but what kind of a message does that send a little girl, as well as any other little boys who may have heard her? That they have to be the same as everybody their own sex? That there are limits on what they can and can't do because of the body they were born with, that they had no control over?

If it seems like I'm harping on a lot about gender in this section, that's because it's one of the most common roots of Social and Personal Rejection. A lot of the criteria we use to judge others are based on gender expectations. That's changing year-by-year. Now, in 2020, they're probably the least prevalent they've been in decades – but they're still an enormous influence on how we judge others, even unconsciously. Gaining an understanding of how you might be enacting those judgements yourself could be a useful tool to find which of *your* behaviours have been brought about by the same pressures.

There's nothing wrong with behaving in a way that conforms to your gender. In fact, there's also nothing wrong with behaving as society thinks you should – as long as it's also how *you* think you should, for your own enjoyment and fulfilment. The problem is that most people think that's what they're doing, and I just don't buy that as many men genuinely love sports/women love fashion as studies claim.

With how complex the human brain is, there's no way so many kids, teenagers and adults would report the same interests as each other... And yet, generally, we boil men and women down to a few acceptable interests. For men, that's sports, cars and chasing women. For women, it's make-up, fashion and being chased by men.

And again, allow me to reiterate – there is *nothing* wrong with behaving in a gender-conforming manner. I personally don't have many feminine interests, and while this is doubtless because I was mainly exposed to masculine hobbies as a child, I feel no repression in choosing to engage with them. Whatever led me to this point, this is who I am and I'm perfectly happy being so. But if you aren't happy acting in the role you are, it might be time for a change.

And, please: if you, in *any way* have control over how younger generations find their own roles, be that as a parent or teacher, give them the freedom to be themselves, free of society's burdens. Don't stop your little boys or girls behaving in ways that don't fit the stereotypes. As long as they're not hurting anybody, who cares? Let them be who they are.

And for that matter, let *yourself* be who you are.

We won't have an authentic society until more of us do.

4
Core Rejection

What is Core Rejection?

And now, the big one. If you read my previous book, you'll already know that my guiding belief is that all men need a clear vision of *what they want* and *who they want to be* in order to feel fulfilled. That's why Core Rejection – rejection of your personal values, guiding beliefs or dreams – is so devastating to a person's well-being.

This isn't like Personal Rejection, where a man might reject his preference for soap operas in favour of whatever the in-vogue car show is. Core Rejection cuts to a much deeper level – it's a rejection of your very *soul,* if you want to get spiritual about it. It most often occurs because you're afraid of ridicule. Core Rejection is the repression of your desire to make a change because you're afraid to rock the boat. It's being too afraid to share what you believe in because other people might call you preachy. At its heart, Core Rejection is rejecting the things you care most about because you're afraid other people won't.

While it can come from a few places, Core Rejection is most often a consequence of Social and Personal Rejection and rarely one of Romantic Rejection. In these cases, it's most often expressed as a tendency to "settle" for something less than you feel you deserve: choosing to stay in a dead-end job because you're afraid of disappointing your friends and family, refusing to chase your dreams in case you disrupt those of your partner...

Core Rejection is often an act of false charity. You do it because you mistakenly believe that helping others means making yourself unhappy. Though that might be true in some cases, it's a dangerous way to live your life. Many people would probably find it *convenient* to be able to walk on top of you when they want to get across a muddy puddle, but that doesn't mean you should stick your face on the ground to please them. Ultimately, if somebody cares about you and you care about them, they should respect your happiness as well as their own. Compromises are made in every relationship, but it's important not to compromise too much of what you truly value.

Unsurprisingly, societal pressures feed into this massively. Gender expectations can play a role here, as it's often seen as unmanly to hold a mission of wanting to help/serve others, but it's also a common issue with those raised in a religious household. I myself was raised an Irish Catholic and rejected my core vision for quite a while out of fear that it wasn't "safe enough" money. (I ended up in retail management instead, worlds apart from personal training/writing.) No one's really looking for "good Christian jobs" or "good Christian relationships" these days, but the values a Christian upbringing instil in us persist.

Core Rejection is the kind of thing that leaves you with deathbed regrets, like the ones we spoke about at the beginning of the book. It's what makes a hundred-year-old wish for a century more so they could live a different life.

Core Rejection is a rejection of purpose, a rejection of your true vision of what you could and should be..

What Does Core Rejection Look Like?

For many, Core Rejection means rejecting what seems like a basic dream – for instance, somebody who dreams of owning their own coffee shop spending years as an office clerk instead. But when you dig deeper, these dreams have an emotional value. That office clerk doesn't just want to own a coffee shop because he likes the smell of coffee. He wants to have a part in making others happy, in providing a safe place for them to retreat to. What he wants is to give value to the world. He may not find this fulfilment in office work – but if you do, then that's great! I'm not judging your career choices. But if a person feels unfulfilled in what they're doing, that's when it's time to make a change.

You might not know what your core desire is. But that doesn't mean you don't have one. Take the time to explore what your core desire might be (as we'll talk about soon) in more abstract terms than the usual "I like to travel/I'd like to own a business." Those may be your real dreams, but they're also an emotional means to an end. Your job is to find out what end you're trying to achieve with them. Find this out and you'll have a much better picture of what truly drives you.

If it's not clear by now, my core desire is to help others become the best version of themselves they can be. My work as a personal trainer is one aspect of this. My writing is another. I want to help men become their best so that they can chase their own desires and be who they truly are without fear of judgement from others. I was unclear about this as a kid, just like everyone else – but over time, the image of the life I wanted became clear to me. Keep an open mind, and the same will happen to you.

We already used the example of the office clerk who wanted to be a barista in the previous paragraph, so let's take a different one.

Imagine that you're working as a receptionist for a computer company. You spend your days answering phones, emailing forms, stapling papers and arranging meetings for your bosses. It's relatively thankless work, but it pays well and you've made friends with everybody in the office. On the surface, there's not too much to be discontent with. A stable job, a steady wage, a pleasant work environment and a short commute.

But what's written on paper doesn't tell the full story.

When you were in university, you chose a Social Care course because you wanted a job that could help the needy and vulnerable. Unfortunately, after graduation, you discovered that jobs in the field are quite limited, and had no choice but to seek office work instead. You worked a few years in data entry before finding a job as a receptionist – and now, 11 years in, the only workplace experience you've got revolves around printing and answering phones, none of which you intended when you went to college.

Circumstances outside of your control, led you into a job you didn't want and made you part of a world you have no interest in. And even though you're not *unhappy* in it, you're... not happy, either.

What you really want is to run your own charity, but you're too afraid to abandon your current job to do so. You know it's what you want to do, but you're not doing it. This is an example of Core Rejection. While you're choosing living the dream life of *somebody else*, somebody else is living yours.

Now, I'm not here to tell you your business – but if I were you, I'd think it was high time to start making moves towards achieving my dream. Without getting too bogged down in the specifics of each situation, the truth is that most "obstacles" to fulfilling your core desire can be worked around... with effort, that is.

If you're so passionate about charity that it was negatively affecting your mental health *not* to work in the field, you could volunteer with one. Part-time work with a cause you care about would probably scratch that itch to help others. Would it take a lot of work? Absolutely. Will it be difficult to juggle another responsibility when you've already got a full-time job? 100%. But does that mean you shouldn't do it? *Hell no.* When you're 100 years old, you won't look back and regret that you juggled jobs to make room for your dream - but you will regret it if you didn't.

That's why, on top of all the psychological reasons not to indulge in Core Rejection, it's also just not *logical* to reject your inner desires. Even if everybody can't achieve the most extreme version of their wildest dreams, we can all pursue elements of them. Nobody can guarantee that you'll become a famous musician... But you can still pick up a guitar and learn to play a few songs (and maybe even write a few of your own).

The same goes for every dream. If all you want is fame for fame's sake, then yeah, it's hard to achieve that. But most of our dreams are a means to an emotional end. So dig deeper into what you want... ask yourself *why* you want it... and discover what you can do *right now* to engage with those desires and experience true fulfilment.

It'd be stupid not to.

How Core Rejection is Internalised

While the internalisation of all forms of rejection leads to self-doubt, self-loathing and cripplingly low self-esteem, Core Rejection is the most damaging kind of all. That's because it's a rejection of your most fundamental desires. The desire to make a change, to find someone who loves you as you are, to be the greatest artist the world has ever seen... these are things that drive us when we have nothing else. By rejecting them, we're rejecting a crucial part of our most basic selves.

To show this, we'll look at the most extreme example of *core rejection:* the deathbed regret. It's a fear many of us, myself included, harbour deep down: the fear that we'll lie on our deathbed and *know,* with chilling certainty, that we should have lived our lives differently. That we should have been kinder, smarter, more diligent. That we should have spent more time with our families. That we should have made a difference in the world.

Few people have deathbed regrets of not saving more. Instead, they regret all the small decisions they made decades before that shaped the futures they went on to live.

Core Rejection is what leads to those regrets. For some, death is the first time they'll ever connect to being alive. But you don't have to let it get that far; you can tackle your deathbed regrets *now,* before you ever get there. You can nip all that pain and suffering in the bud if you learn to see yourself honestly, accept yourself fully and act in accordance with your core beliefs.

To contrast Core Rejection further with the other forms, let's look again at the description I gave at the beginning of the book. This is a good way to show how your subconscious internalises each form.

Social rejection: *"There is something wrong with the way I act."* ***(How you're judged by society at large)***

Romantic rejection: *"There is something wrong with who/what I am."* ***(How you're judged by people you're interested in romantically)***

Personal rejection: *"There's something wrong with my interests."* ***(How you judge yourself for the things you're interested in and the ways you behave)***

Core rejection: *"There's something wrong with my existence."* ***(How you judge yourself for your core desires/vision)***

If understanding your core desire goes a little like this:

"I want to run my own coffee shop." → *"I want to serve others."* → *"I want to provide a safe place for people."*

OR

"I want to run my own charity." → *"I want to do good in the world."* → *"I want to provide for the needy."*

Then *rejecting* your core desire looks more like:

"I want to provide a safe place for people, but that dream is too hard to achieve." → *"I'm going to focus on something more sensible instead."* → *"My dream isn't sensible or worth pursuing."* → *"What I want isn't worth pursuing."* → *"My personal desires aren't important."*

OR

"Even though I want to work in charity, I'm going to keep my office job." → "Keeping this job is more responsible than following my purpose." → "Being responsible is more important than being true to myself." → "Being true to myself isn't important." → "My personal desires aren't important."

Because we define ourselves internally by the things we *want*, believing our desires don't matter has the exact same effect as believing that *we* don't matter. Unlike romantic and social rejection (which can be "cured" through positive social and romantic experiences), the self-loathing brought on by core rejection is impossible to tackle without acting on the rejected desires. This isn't easy; but there's a reason I called *Core Rejection* "the big one" at the start of this section.

Human beings are vision given form. Vision is what drives us; it runs in our veins. Without a clear vision, success and happiness will never be attainable. Core Rejection is internalised as rejection of vision, and so getting past it is crucial to becoming stronger.

There are many paths to doing so - some of which will be outlined and explored in the following section - but introspection is a mandate for all of them. Sorry to say it, but if you historically don't like to think about your feelings, you're just going to have to get over it. Nobody heals by ignoring a wound. And particularly in the case of Core Rejection, which so many of us suffer from without ever being aware of it... it's important that you take the time to look inwards.

In this process, you may discover that some things you *thought* were core desires, actually aren't. You might learn that something you've always dreamed of having was actually a cover for something else, something that'll truly fulfil you. There's no certainty with this. That's what makes it scary. But at the end of the process, you'll be better equipped to live an authentic life.

- To become the strongest you can be, you first need a strong foundation.

- To have a strong foundation, you must understand who you are at your core.

- To understand who you are at your core, you need to understand your core desires.

- And to understand your core desires, you need to discover and process the elements of them, which you've been rejecting.

The process could be instantaneous - or it could be the longest, most drawn-out task of your life. There's a reason it takes some people so long to *find themselves*, after all. But in either case, the time you spend will prove to be worthwhile.

You'll see as much, once you've experienced *core acceptance* for yourself.

5

Healing From Rejection

For those of you, who skipped ahead to this point, allow me this space to plead that you read the book the whole way through. No single form of rejection is completely disconnected from the rest - even if you just came here for tips on getting past a break-up, reading about the other forms can be beneficial to your understanding of elements that may have led to your breakup or teach you how to understand others better. That being said, you're free to do what you want with a book you paid for: so let's get this show on the road.

Now, before we get started:

I think it's important to clarify that I won't be discussing specific tactics for getting over each type of rejection in this part of the book. Since I already wrote about the specifics of social/romantic/personal/core rejection in each of their respective chapters, I won't be writing a section called "Top 10 Breakup Tips" here. I'd just be wasting your time. The truth is that "getting over" rejection is the same as "getting over" any kind of emotional pain - and selling you snake-oil tactics for coping with friends being mean/your spouse misunderstanding you, just distracts from that.

The kind of healing I'm going to talk about isn't glamorous. It's not quick, easy or fun. But it's effective and it's time-tested by many more than just me. Approach it with an open mind and you'll be surprised how much it can help you.

And with that...

For as bad as I've made rejection sound throughout this book, it's not all doom and gloom. Rejection is a valuable teaching tool for how to better interact with others/ yourself, and can be a powerful mechanism for growth when used correctly. It hurts to be rejected, no matter the reason - but like how the stress of lifting heavy weights triggers muscle growth, the damage rejection causes can be used to build you back up stronger than before.

The only problem is that this doesn't happen naturally for most of us. As social, tribe-driven animals, we thrive on acceptance. Rejection is the worst-case scenario to our lizard brains. Rejection was like Armageddon for the cavemen, and our brains don't understand natively that it's not quite so big a deal now. Rejection is naturally internalised as a wound... and like all wounds, it festers if left untreated.

So then the question becomes not how you *heal* from rejection, but how you *treat* it. That might seem like much of a muchness, but they're two very different angles to approach the subject from.

The only thing that will *heal* rejection is time. Distance from the time of injury is needed to close an ego wound; no guru, meditation or pill will do that for you, try as companies might to convince you they will. Some can speed up the healing process, of course, but that number's far lower than what's on the market.

In my eyes, there are two keys to speeding up recovery from rejection/ensuring that it's internalised as something *useful* rather than plain damage.

Those are:

1. Introspection/meditation/reflection/whatever else fits the bill of bringing *awareness* to your pain. This will enable you to understand why/how rejections have hurt you

2. Learning to re-contextualise/change your perspective on rejection so that it can be processed as something *beneficial* instead of just damaging

But you won't have to figure out how to do this by yourself. For starters, if you've read the book closely up until now, you'll probably already have begun to understand how rejection can be reframed as a positive or at least how it can be seen as *less negative.* As a refresher, here are some quick-and-dirty insights on why each kind of rejection isn't really worth dwelling on.

Why It's Not Worth Dwelling On: Social Rejection

Since platonic rejection by peers, colleagues, employers and family members so often stems from societal expectations, recognising the hypocrisy of those expectations takes the sting out of it. By now, I hope you've gained an understanding of why the "shoulds" of society are a terrible barometer to live your life by. But if you haven't...

1. It's ridiculous to prescribe *one set way of life* to half the world's population and a different one to the other half. We're all individuals with individual needs, tastes and desires. Anybody who rejects you for not fitting their binary views of what men/women are/aren't "supposed" to do is an idiot.

2. Same goes for anybody who rejects you based on your race/apparent ethnicity. As harsh as it sounds, you're better off without them. *Bye-bye!*

3. And as for rejections based on your class/economic status... well, I think the stupidity of this one goes without saying.

It's a different story if you're being socially rejected because you've done something hurtful. But assuming you've done your best to be a decent person and aren't actively hurting others, it means nothing. Shake it off and move on.

Why It's Not Worth Dwelling On: Romantic Rejection

For starters, any romantic rejection that comes from someone you're not in a relationship with (i.e. someone you're hitting on) is 100% based on external factors, such as appearance or fashion. It obviously hurts to be shot down when approaching someone you fancy but it's important to remember that:

A. Everybody's got different taste.

One person's "no" is another person's "yes".

B. They're making the rejection based on *their* value system and *their* expectations of their partners.

It says a lot more about you than it does them.

It still hurts to be shot down, especially if it's based on factors of your appearance you have no control over. But don't take one or two rejections as evidence of what'll happen on the 10th, 50th or 100th. Everyone's attractive to somebody... and I do mean *everyone.* If you think oth-erwise, remember - the only reason an "ugly" person can even exist nowadays is that their "ugly" ancestors have spent thousands of years reproducing.

Chin up. Stay confident. You'll be fine.

Admittedly, rejection from somebody you're actually *in* a relationship with is a little different. But since it's probably fair to say that *most* romantic rejection is an emotional response vs. a societal one, we can still break partner rejections into two broad categories.

A. Your partner's reasoning is unfair or misguided.

They dump you over something that didn't happen/ wasn't your true intention, because they were bored, because they found someone new... in any case where a partner's rejection is genuinely *not* due to your actions, the fault for it ultimately lies with them. They're the one being disrespectful, and you're the one in the position to decide whether you even want to move forward or not. Disentangling any guilt you feel for the breakup, will help you to see that and move on.

B. Your partner's reasoning is fair and accurate.

They're breaking up with you because you *have* wronged them, you *were* a bad partner and you both know it. Anyone who breaks up with you for a reason you agree with is doing you a favour. They're offering a rare opportunity for growth by exposing a flaw in yourself that you might have never seen otherwise. You might not be able to salvage your current relationship, but you can use the pain of this kind of breakup to make you a better person and partner for whoever comes next. You'll find love again.

And if the rejection in question isn't relationship-ending, then use it to become a better version of yourself. Don't let the baggage of past hurts stop you from growing into the man you know you can be. Face up to your shortcomings. Do the work. Fix yourself, then watch your relationship improve in turn.

Why It's Not Worth Dwelling On: Personal And Core Rejection

Both these types of rejections are rejections of desire.

Personal Rejection is the rejection of surface-level personality traits, usually done to appease the whims of a group (friends/family/colleagues) or partner.

Core Rejection is an individual's rejection of their core vision, usually done because of low self-esteem or self-worth.

Both are painful. Both are fuelled by pressures from the outside world. But both forms can be treated by *direct action,* and the emotional hurt they cause can be helped by understanding this one thing.

The only life worth living is the one that makes you WANT to be alive.

Don't let fear stop you from engaging with who you really are. Don't let society shame you into choosing hobbies you don't care about, and don't let friends/family push you away from your dreams. At the end of the day, Personal and Core Rejection are optional, both choices a person makes based on feedback from the outside world.

But which do you think you'll regret more on your deathbed - letting those outside voices tell you how you're allowed to live or working to seize the life you want?

It won't ever be any less scary to think about. But you just need the courage to take that first step towards living authentically: once you do, the rest will come naturally.

Take the time to read through those points again if you're still unsure of what we've covered so far. Once you're sure you're comfortable with them, you're ready to begin the next step: healing the hurt of past rejections. To start with, let's run through some exercises to help you understand the kinds of wounds rejection leaves.

The Most Important Test You'll Ever Take

I've mentioned it before in this book and my last one, that precise reflection and self-awareness are undoubtedly two of the most important skills any person can have. Understanding who you are and more importantly *how* you came to be that person, are vital to achieving fulfilment.

In the context of this book, I'd like you to focus your attention on the rejections you've experienced in the course of your life - how they happened, why they happened and how you internalised them. To do this, I'd like you to set some time aside, pick up a pencil/pen and answer the following questions into whatever notebook you can find. (Please, don't do this on any page scraps. It's way too important to risk losing.)

If you take the time to answer these questions sincerely, it may well be the Most Important Test You'll Ever Take. The answers will do much more than get you into college or let you drive a car; they'll show you a way through the pain of rejection and connect you with your truest self.

So, let's get started!

Getting to Grips With Rejection

Q1: If I ask you to think of a rejection you experienced outside of the last seven days, what rejection comes to mind?

____

____

Q2: What was your relationship with the person who made this rejection? Were they your spouse? Classmate? Manager?

____

____

Q3: If you can, turn your attention to your memory of the event. (This might be painful, but it's important you follow through with it.) List the sensations you can remember of the event, if any. How did being rejected like that make you feel in the moment? How was the rejection processed physically?

Q4: How long would you estimate (this can be a rough guess!) it took you to get over the initial sting of the rejection? In other words, how long did it take for those sensations listed above to fade?

Q5: When those physical sensations did fade, were you then emotionally at peace with the rejection? Or did the psychological effects outlast the physical ones? (Hint: the answer to the first half of this should be no, and the answer to the second half should be yes. If you've answered differently, think carefully about whether or not you're being honest with yourself.)

Q6: How long did it take for the emotional sting of the rejection to fade, if it did at all?

Q7: How was your relationship with the rejecter affected by this rejection? You should answer this from two perspectives: first think about how it was affected in the immediate aftermath, and then about how it was affected once the first sting of it had faded.

Q8: If your answer differed from each perspective, what do you think happened to change your emotional response to the rejecter?

Q9: Has the rejection had a permanent impact on the way you view the rejecter?

____

____

Q10: Does thinking about the rejection still make you uncomfortable/guilty/upset on some level?

____

____

If your answer to the last question is a genuine, heartfelt *no*, congratulations! You've probably exorcised the rejection in your own way, and have escaped negatively internalising it. But if you're anything like me (and if you've read this far in the book, you probably are!) then the answer to Q10 will be a resounding *yes.* Even if the flutter of negativity is weak, it still counts - if you feel any ill-will towards yourself or another when you think about the rejection, that shows you're still holding that bad feeling in your body.

Too often, we mistake the physical manifestations of emotion as our internal experience of them - we believe that because our eyes and back no longer feel tight, our tension must be gone, or that the fact we're not crying about something means we can't be sad. But even though there's a strong connection between our psychological and physical selves, they're worlds apart when it comes to healing and recovery. Crying is the best example of this. When we finish crying (and if it's been a while since you have, think back to the last instance you remember), we feel a sense of physical relief and catharsis. Crying's a great way to externalise negative emotion; its positive effects are numerous and well-recorded in both scientific journals and literature.

As French writer Antoine de Rivarol once said (in French, of course):

> *"Heavy hearts, like heavy clouds in the sky, are best relieved by the letting of a little water."*

But when you think back to the last time you cried, is it true that you felt 100% better when you were finished? You might have felt significant improvement - but was it *total* improvement?

(Spoiler alert: it wasn't.)

The residual negativity left after that process might not feel significant - you might argue that if 98% of the sadness/pain is gone, what does the last 2% matter? - but those residual numbers add up over time. If the physical injuries you sustain only *mostly* healed, you'd be riddled with aches and pains by the time you hit your 20s. Emotional hurts work like that. The final 2% of hundreds of rejections, self-directed or otherwise, add up over time into negative habits and toxic thought patterns. They shape the way you view yourself and your relationships with others. They limit how you trust, influence how you behave and ultimately manifest as issues of body image, self-esteem and bouts of self-loathing.

It's not possible to fully eliminate all past hurts. Some things, no matter how much time you give them, will always hurt to think about. Grief will always be grief. Betrayal will always be betrayal. Only time can ease the impact of emotional wounds that severe, and there's a limit to how effective even time can be. But the other, lesser hurts you bottle up? They can be dealt with. There's no need for a stern talking-to by your primary school teacher to tear you up inside or for the girlfriend who cheated on you when you were 15 to affect your relationships today.

Which brings me to the initial aim of this section: to help you *understand* how your hurts have shaped you, and then *reframe* those hurts as steps towards a better life. Reframing life's random, chaotic cruelties as chances for positive change is a good way to take the historical sting out of them. It'll help you bounce back from future rejections quicker, too.

The questions above helped you gain an understanding of the physicality and internalisation of rejections, but the next exercise will help you learn how rejection has shaped your personality.

How Rejection Has Shaped Your Personality

Q1: If I ask you to think of the *earliest* example of rejection you can remember, what event comes to mind?

____

____

Q2: What was your relationship to the rejecter in this instance? (Odds are, if it's from childhood, it won't be an employer.)

____

____

Q3: Why do you think this rejection stuck in your mind? Were you punished for it in a memorable way, etc., or was your emotional response so significant that you can't help but remember it?

Q4: What do you think this rejection taught you at the time? / What do you think this rejection was *meant* to teach you at the time? (This could be something as simple as "don't snack before dinner" or "don't interrupt Mammy when she's working" or as complex as "you're not worth as much as your sister." Write whatever answer comes to mind.)

Q5: Do you think this rejection was effective as a lesson? Why/why not?

____

____

Q6: In hindsight, did this rejection affect your behaviour afterwards?

____

____

Q7: If you answered yes to Q6, how was your behaviour affected?

____

____

Q8: Taking inspiration from the examples of internalisation listed earlier in the book (i.e. “rejection” → “alleged fact” → “internalisation”) how do you think you internalised this particular rejection?

____

____

Q9: Do you feel that this change in behaviour had an impact on choices you made in situations separate from the rejecter? (i.e. if you were harshly scolded for interrupting your father while he was on the phone, were you more cautious when other people were on the phone in future?)

Q10: Ultimately, do you think this rejection was *fair* and had a *net positive* effect on your behaviour?

Q11: Ultimately, do you think this rejection was *kind* and had a *net positive* effect on your psychology? (The answers to Q10 and Q11 can be different.)

(If some of those questions were tricky, don't worry about it - abstract questions like Q8/Q11 are meant to be challenging. Learning new ways to explore emotion means learning new thought patterns. Like learning anything new, there's bound to be a bit of a learning curve. Even if it feels unnatural at first, just answer them as best you can. There is no *right* or *wrong* way to self-reflect.)

The answers to these questions will all be illuminating, but those of Q8, Q9 and Q11 should be of particular interest to you. These are the questions that show how rejection can shape your future feelings/behaviours. (Of course, there's always the possibility that you believe this rejection had zero impact on you, but... again, if you're anything like me, that's really very unlikely. If you answered as such, make sure you're being honest with yourself. If you are, go buy an ice cream or something. You're clearly too emotionally well-rounded for me to do anything with.)

Taking the mundane example of, again, being scolded for interrupting a parent's phone call, let's look at how this might impact your behaviour in the immediate aftermath.

There are three likely possibilities:

A. You might be fearful of that parent for the next few hours or so, until either their temper or your hurt has cooled.

B. You might try to make amends with them in some way.

C. You might be *so offended* that you attempt to take revenge by annoying them in some other way.

Whatever choice you make right then, will impact future interactions with the parent. But outside of the immediate aftermath, your behaviour is shaped by the rejections you accrue over the course of your life.

After such a rejection, you might:

A. Go out of your way to avoid the parent in question when they're on the phone. (A fear response.)

B. Learn and respect the need for silence when somebody's on the phone. (A corrective response, likely what the parent intends.)

C. Carry on with the previous behaviour until another rejection like this occurs and the cycle of decision/ consequence begins again. (A failure to internalise the rejection in any way, either positive or negative.)

These are the behavioural impacts of such a rejection. More than likely, you'll internalise the rejection with a corrective response and learn not to interrupt people when they're on the phone. But what's interesting about even a rejection as simple as this, is how profound an impact it has on a person's actions. The first time you're taught not to interrupt people when they're on the phone probably occurs during childhood - but it's something you'll remember forever, even into adulthood. Such is the power of social rejection - it teaches us the rules of interaction in a way that's impossible to forget.

But aside from its benefits, the emotional impacts of social rejection can be extremely damaging. This isn't to say that this single instance will shred a child's self-esteem or emotional wellbeing; provided you're not an absolute tool about it, there's no reason they should even be that upset. But emotionally vulnerable children (AKA, sensitive kids) can internalise the accrued negativity of such rejections as comments on their worth/place in society on a subconscious level, and this will shape how they interact with others going forward. If you disagree with that statement, let me ask you: why did you remember the specific example of rejection you wrote about above?

(Spoiler alert, again: *it's because you remember the emotional impact it had on you.*)

Small rejections, over time, are like an ego death by a thousand cuts. Most people can shrug them off - but everyone has little quirks that stem from rejections like these, no matter how minor they may seem.

The way they knock before entering a room. The way they always double-check that the door is locked. Even the way they throw/catch things; all small quirks shaped by brief instances of social rejection, behaviours adapted to avoid negative response from others. (As a bonus exercise, see if you can think of some rejections that might inspire these behaviours/quirks!)

Ultimately, *personality* is just a fancy word for "how we interact with the world." Our quirks and behaviours *are* our external personalities and since rejection is what shapes those... rejection is what shapes our personalities. It teaches us to act more politely, be more withdrawn, feel more timid, etc. Most of the time, social rejection is meant to shape us into more "acceptable" members of society. As we discussed earlier in the book, that concept's a little nonsensical and a poor reason for emotional upset... but it's not explicitly damaging.

Social rejection is what first taught our selfish, greedy selves kindness when we were kids. Goodness is a social act; I'm sure we all know people who only act good/polite so that others will *think* they're good/polite. And since hypocritical politeness is important to prevent the crumbling of civilisation, that's probably OK in the long run. The problem is that social rejection *also* teaches us that we have to reject our desires.

We don't just learn to ignore our *selfish* desires when we're scolded as children. At that age, we've got no concept of what it means to be self*ish* vs. self*less.* So instead of hearing "don't indulge selfish desires" (which is not a message a 5-year old will understand), kids hear "don't indulge *your* desires."

Some kids won't be adversely affected by this. Others will. The affected ones grow up repressing their true selves and get so good at rejecting their core desires that they almost convince themselves of their happiness. But, in the end, they'll learn too that what they've got is somebody *else's* ideal life. Not their own.

It's nobody's fault that rejection manifests like this. It's not *wrong* to teach your kids good manners, no more so than it is for an employer to discipline their staff. I've done both in my time and there's no use feeling guilty for the hurt I *might* have caused - especially since most of them won't have thought much of it. But for the ones who do... the ones who grew up feeling rejected, who are *used* to their self-image being defined by others' disappointment... it's important that they (we) learn to process their emotions in a healthy way.

Which brings us to the million-dollar question.

How do You Heal From Rejection?

You've done the exercises. You've discovered all your repressed childhood traumas (you're welcome, by the way). You've got a clear image in your head of how the rejections of your youth, adolescence and even recent adulthood have shaped your behaviours and consequently, your personality.

So now how do you make it hurt less?

The answer is simple. Not fun, not by any stretch of the imagination - but it's definitely simple to execute. Emotional pain, like any negative stimulus, needs two things from you in order to heal.

#1: Attention

#2: Time

#1 The First Ingredient: Attention

Think of emotional pain like a super bright light and your mind as a dark room. When you first look at the light, your eyes are going to hurt a bit - but as your pupils adjust to the new amount of light in the room, that pain will fade. You'll still be able to recognise that it's bright, but that alone won't be a problem for you. You'll adjust to it.

Dealing with emotional pain is like looking at a bright light. It'll hurt at first - and maybe it'll always hurt a little, if you've got sensitive eyes - but it'll get exponentially easier to handle if you expose yourself to it. It'll take time and it'll take focused attention and reflection... but eventually, the pain will lessen.

Note: A Word on Mental Health Professionals

Without going into too much detail, since it's just not my story to tell, I've got more experience with this than I care to admit. Years ago, I was involved in a car accident that was fatal for the other driver. I had a lot of trouble getting past, and I sought therapy to help me through it. I'm not going to say I *ended up* getting help as if it's some rock bottom, because it isn't. Mental pain is different to physical pain, but the healing process is quite similar. Just like some cuts heal on their own while others need stitches, some mental issues might need more assistance than others.

Whatever advice I give in this segment, know that therapy is always an option if you're finding it tough to get past something. Therapists nowadays do a lot more than "just listen" to their patients, though they do that too. Cognitive-behavioural therapists teach skills and coping mechanisms that ease the struggle of the healing process. Holistic, at-home remedies are all well and good... but some problems need more care than meditation and journalling can give.

And it's OK to seek it.

Bringing Awareness To The Problem

There are multiple ways to bring attention to emotional pain. The questions listed a few pages back can be one: depending on the emotions they dredge up, you could use them as a shortcut to analyse how you feel about a particular rejection. But if that's not enough, I'd recommend journalling as the next home-remedy. *Proper* journalling, mind you, not glorified To-Do listing. Give yourself an A4 page, an hour and a topic of hurt and let the words flow. Even if you're not much of a writer, giving yourself and your pain an unbridled train of release is a great way to bring attention to any hurt you hold.

You might have the instinct to flinch away from this task. But it's crucial to your development that you embrace the challenge this presents. Looking at your problems *written out* can make you feel all sorts of emotions, and practicing total surrender to them is an excellent way to learn new coping skills. Guilt, anger, fear... it doesn't matter what, just let yourself feel it in its totality.

Once you've done that, depending on the kind of rejection you're reflecting on, you should leave it a few days and then re-read that train of thought. (Getting some distance from what you've written is important for this.) Reading it will probably hurt as much as writing it - but this time, pick through what you've written to see if it really makes sense. Are the feelings you've expressed rooted in reality or in someone else's opinion of it?

This is where you'll need to explore the illogic of letting rejection control the way you feel. Taking inspiration from the examples in earlier sections of how your mind processes the judgements of others, search your writing for places where you've done the same. (Again, it goes something like "rejection" → "alleged fact" → "internalisation") If you've written about how much you've been hurt by a recent break-up or divorce, there'll probably be some untrue "*I am*" statements in there. "*I am worthless*", "*I am totally at fault*", "*I am never going to find love*"... these are great places to practice this technique on.

Working backwards from your internalisation of a rejection, you'll be able to see the gaps in your emotional logic much more clearly. Is it really fair to say that, because your boss scolded you for being late, *everybody* in your office hates you? Do you honestly believe, with 100% certainty, that being passed over for a wedding invitation means your friends are pretending to like you?

Probably not. But that's the meaning your subconscious extracts from a negative emotional event. It all goes back to the tribal psychology we discussed in the first chapter. We're so desperate to belong that we'll do anything to avoid rejection... no matter how bad it is for ourselves. But turning external rejection (social rejection, romantic rejection) to internal (personal rejection, core rejection) isn't a foregone conclusion. The better you get at finding the discrepancies in your pain, the less rejections will hurt in future.

In the end, *awareness* is what'll protect you from hurt. Getting familiar with your pain is the only way to ease it.

But if journalling *really* isn't your thing, you can always try meditation. I'm sure I don't need to explain what it is to you, but just in case you've been living under a rock for the last ten years... When I say meditation, I'm not referring to levitating like a monk or incessant chanting of mantras. I'm talking about a period of silence and stillness a person carves out in their day, where they can bring full attention to all the sensations of their inner world.

For many people, meditation begins with finding a seat in a quiet place. They close their eyes; they begin to breathe more deeply; and over the next 10, 15, 20 minutes or so, they count their breaths. You should try it whenever you get a chance - even two minutes is a good starting point. Focus on nothing but the sensation of breath and the mental counting of breaths in and out and let all other thoughts pass you by.

Meditation is about training your attention. Whenever you lose count of your breaths or feel yourself beginning to daydream, just bring that attention back to the breath and begin the count again. It sounds easy, but you'd be surprised how much you'll lose count of breaths at first. In the digital age, our focus is scattered by default. Our attention spans are shrinking. But meditation is a way to counteract that - and once you're familiar with the practice of quietly breathing and counting, you can use the process to explore your emotions instead.

This is a little more abstract than "writing your thoughts on paper", which is why it's not what I recommend first...

but you can achieve the same results by replaying memories of rejections and checking your emotional response the same way you'd check your written train of thought. *Why does X make me feel Y, is it fair that I interpreted that as Z,* etc.

#2 The Second Ingredient: Time

Whatever method of introspection you choose, this isn't a task you can complete in a day. It could take a few weeks of practice for this to pay off - especially since, if you're wise, you won't try to tackle all your rejection-based traumas in one sitting. Taking it slow is not only recommended, it's *required* if you want proper healing. No matter how good a doctor is, there's no changing how quick your body mends a broken bone. The doctor can give you a cast, sure. They can provide physiotherapy, massage, prescribe rest and medication and vitamins... but the bone's going to heal at its own pace.

Emotional hurt heals the same, regardless of whether you've been injured by rejection or something else entirely, like grief. Like the doctor who prescribes rest and massage, all you can do is ensure your mental foundation is solid for recovery. It doesn't matter how emotionally intelligent or well-adjusted you are: rejection will always sting, grief will always ache and hurt will find a way through any walls of denial you build inside. That's why *attention* and *time* must be taken in tandem. Attention opens a window for trapped hurt to escape through, but that doesn't make it move any faster.

Of course, not all rejection is created equal. Some hurts heal quicker than others. It's easier to get over being snubbed by an acquaintance vs. a friend or having your advances spurned by a stranger vs. a partner. Also, some people just feel rejection less than others. Personally, I don't think I've ever been hit hard by societal judgements. Even as a kid, being told I "should" act a certain way because I was a boy didn't bother me.

But on the other hand, getting past my core rejection of what I truly wanted in life took a lot of work. We all have different tolerances for different kinds of rejection... but as a rule, the less internalised a rejection is, the quicker the hurt heals. That's why it's important to learn how your subconscious internalises rejection - being aware of the process will stop it from happening.

Most of us are pretty bad at this at first. We take everything personally, even if we think we don't. We draw deep meaning from inane rejection, and use the judgements of others to define how we feel about ourselves. We allow society to tell us that we're wrong for being who we are. We let friends decide how we should look, act and think. We water our personalities down so much for our partners, there's hardly anything distinctive left in us at all. Rejections rooted in childhood and important developmental relationships (i.e. your first love, favourite teachers, close friends) are the hardest to heal, as they cut the deepest... but attention and time will (mostly) heal pretty much anything.

Exercise kindness. Treat your emotional self like a sad friend or partner; be supportive, not forceful. Don't call yourself *stupid* or *weak* for the things that hurt you. It doesn't matter how inane it seems. Your feelings are valid and should be treated as such. Give yourself the time and space you need to recover. Regardless of how long it takes - it could be years or it could be hours - remember to *stay the course.* Confronting your rejections head on is the best way to kill the pain they cause. Even if it takes longer than you'd like for the pain to fade, you'll be getting stronger every time you feel it... and over time, it'll hurt less and less.

You've just got to be patient.

Moving On Without Fear

The sad reality of rejection is that it never stops hurting. Old rejections always sting a little. New ones always burn. But it's your choice whether or not to let pain dictate how you live your life.

All rejection is *supposed* to be corrective.

Social Rejection *corrects* you into being a more acceptable member of society.

Romantic Rejection *corrects* you into changing your behaviour or finding a new partner.

The self-directed **Personal Rejection** *corrects* you into more conventional interests/behaviours, to decrease the chance of peer rejection.

Core Rejection *corrects* you into living a safer life, at the cost of an extraordinary one.

But you know as well as I do that these corrections are misguided. Even *if* following every single one let you live a more acceptable life, there's no guarantee that'll make you happy. In fact, it's probably going to do the opposite. Being forced to suppress your desires, the big and the small, is just going to make you miserable.

That's why living authentically, in accordance to *your* desires, is so important. It's why you have to keep going in the face of rejection. If you let the judgement of others knock you off your own path, you'll end up on a road you never wanted that leads to a destination you never asked for.

Be kind. Be honest. Strive to be the best you can be, and treat others as respectfully as you'd want to be treated. Once you know you're doing that, no rejection will ever matter again. As long as you're a good person, you're allowed your quirks and odd behaviours, even the ones that don't make sense to most people.

If you need permission for that, then I'll be the one to give it to you. *I hereby declare* that you're free to be who you want to be and *do* what you want, as long as you're not hurting anyone.

Rejection hurts because of what we make of it, not because of what it *is.* It hurts because we internalise the rejection of others as rejection of ourselves, and use outside approval as a metric of life success. It stings to be shot down in a club because we interpret it as proof that we don't deserve or will never find love; it stings to be passed over for a promotion because we take it to mean that we don't deserve anything better than what we have. Learning to overcome your distorted thoughts (subconscious or otherwise) is what will ultimately make rejection hurt less and retroactively let old rejections begin to heal.

Have faith in the process. Have faith in yourself! And remember that no matter what kind of rejection you're dealing with... no matter where it's coming from or why... dealing with that hurt will only make you stronger.

That's what'll enable you to live your authentic life.

6

Lessons Learned Along The Way

Through my personal journey of self-acceptance, I've learned some valuable life lessons. In these chapters, I'll share them with you. Consider them a P.S to the rest of the book... or a bonus, I guess, since they're not explicitly about rejection! My hope is that they'll help you avoid making the same mistakes I have, or even just help you understand what you're going through a little better.

Either way, I hope you enjoy the following insights.

Lesson One: Take Responsibility

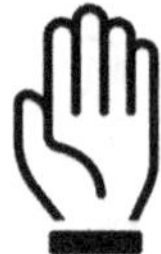

Sounds basic - but you'd be surprised how many adults struggle with this.

Or, maybe you wouldn't. You might have friends or a partner or grown-up kids who still act a little too much like teenagers for their own good. Maybe they blame all their problems on other people, or adopt a woe-is-me attitude towards the world to avoid having to take any action themselves.

(Or, if you're anything like me... maybe you were/are that person yourself, at one time or another.)

A key part of adulthood is learning to take responsibility for your own actions. At its core, it's a concept that's widely espoused in primary education. Teaching kids what their *responsibilities* are to themselves and the wider society is a crucial part of development. But what's spoken about less often is the parallel importance of agency and personal choice, and how only the responsibilities **you** choose to take and accept will be of any real value to you.

In psychology, there's a concept called the *locus of control* that defines how much a person feels they can control their lives. If a person has an internal locus of control, they have a mental belief that they can make things happen - and therefore, that they control their own futures. The opposite is an external locus of control, where a person feels powerless to affect change in their own lives. They believe they've got no agency in their own lives, and that they've got no control over what happens to them.

If you're anything like me, you probably have the following quote from Shakespeare's "The Merchant of Venice" burned into your head since you were 15 years old:

***"I hold the world but as the world, Gratiano;
a stage where every man must play a part,
and mine a sad one."***

We all know someone who sees life like this - as a stage where we're all bound to play specific roles, stuck with lines we've got no say over. This attitude is obviously negative, and so we roll our eyes when we come across it... but it's not just personal problems this attitude handwaves away. People who believe they've got no agency also believe they've got no personal responsibility for their actions, and that they can't be held accountable for them. *It's not my fault I cheated on you,* they argue. *It's because I was raised wrong. It's because someone hurt me. Can't you see it's the world's fault? You have to take me back!*

But that idea's bullshit. Voluntary actions are, by definition, *voluntary.* No matter what influences your choices, you're still personally responsible for them.

We've all got control over our lives. Sure, you might be "stuck" in a dead-end job or relationship or a crappy financial situation or with debilitating health issues... and all of these, understandably, can make you feel like life's out of your control. But that's true for everyone. We're all bound by the laws of nature, if nothing else; gravity, the aging process, mortality. But why let the removal of a few choices strip you of the rest? You should want to be in charge of yourself. You should *want* to take active choice in your life! You're more than an actor in someone else's production. No matter what limitations you face, you have to take responsibility for what you can - for what *you know you can* - and make your life your own.

Nobody else will do that for you.

Lesson Two: Build Momentum, Then Keep Going

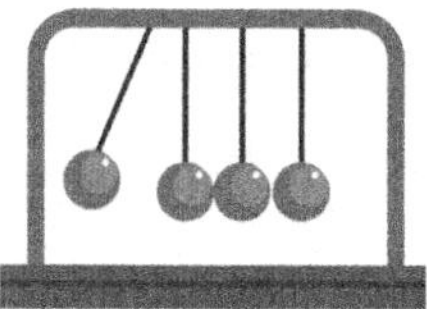

Getting stuff done is hard, some days more than others. I wake up some mornings and wish I could sleep another sixteen hours... but I'm a grown up, so instead, I count to three and throw the covers off. That way, I have to move or else I'll get cold.

(#lifehacks)

Motivation and decision-making are some of the most-talked about topics in the self-improvement world. As I write this, a dozen books on the subject are floating to mind, books many would say are the key to *changing your life forever*. And honestly, they might be... but that doesn't mean they're unique. Most of them just contain the information I'm about to write in the next few paragraphs, but stretched out across 50,000+ words. You probably know most of it already, too. This probably isn't the first book of the genre you've read... but even assuming you're familiar with it, my hope is that this'll remind you to put the content into practice.

The decisions we make on an everyday basis take varying amounts of energy/willpower/discipline, depending on what they are. Getting up when you're tired and it's cold outside takes a lot more energy than getting up when you're well-rested. Going for a run or working out takes more activation energy than watching TV. Because humans are fundamentally lazy creatures (you don't see monkeys lifting weights, do you?), we tend to take the path of least resistance. We want to choose the tasks with the lowest activation energy because... well, it's easier.

But here's the kicker: how difficult it is to start doing something says nothing about how beneficial it will be to you.

This is true in both directions. It's technically easy to eat a salad, and probably takes less effort than deep-frying a chicken, but it's much healthier for you. And on the flipside, while it'd be *difficult* to run in circles for six hours, that doesn't mean it'll benefit you. It's not quite accurate to say that a task's value is calculable based on how difficult it is - not everything "challenging" is worth the effort. It's important to recognise that and to learn to evaluate the pros/cons of any action *separately* from its difficulty. A literal pros-and-cons list can be a good way to do this. If you're struggling to start a task, write down what you'd like to do instead and then compare the benefits and drawbacks of both. This should help give some perspective on which is worth spending your time on.

But Gavin, I hear you say. *I know I should go for a run, but it's just so much effort! I can't make myself do it. It's too hard!*

(Feel free to sub in your actual thoughts in place of the above. My ability to read minds tends to break down over long distances.)

It's a valid point. Starting hard tasks is... well, hard. But while most books devolve here into "hacks" that make starting a task easier, ranging from "drink a coffee" to "bathe in the blood of your enemies", I'll just ask you a question.

What's the smallest amount of the task you CAN do?

If it's going for a run you're struggling with, can you put on your running shoes? Can you tie them? If that's literally all you can do, then do that - seriously. No shame here.

And once that's done, can you make yourself run for five seconds? And another five? And how about another five after that?

Momentum is an underrated component of action, but it's probably the easiest way to "make" yourself do something hard. If you're struggling with the idea of exercising for an hour, forget about the hour. How about doing just the first five seconds of it? Sounds easier, right? Almost pointlessly so - but if you can take any task five seconds at a time, you'll be able to reach the end of it.

By breaking a task into its smallest parts and taking them on one-by-one, you're giving yourself the best possible chance of success. The momentum of completing each small step will carry you onto the next - and I don't need any studies to back that up. I'm sure you've seen it yourself. Ever been out walking somewhere and you got so tired that you've had to focus on moving one foot at a time? Ever been faced with a difficult exam or aptitude test that you've had to break into tiny, manageable segments for your own sanity? This works because momentum is king. It's hard to get going - but once we do that, it gets easier to stay that way. The amount of energy required to maintain an action is significantly less than the amount required to start it, because *momentum* takes over and carries us forward.

This is true in a micro and macro sense. Days that start off well keep going well; days that don't start well usually go off-track. To illustrate this point, here's a simple example from my own life.

As of the time of writing, I've been going for an early morning swim in the ocean every day for the past month. Some days, it's the last thing in the world I want to do. Honestly, I'd usually rather sleep in than face those cold waves. On days where I really struggle, I do exactly what I talk about above. I don't think about splashing around in freezing water for 45 minutes while I'm lying in bed. Instead, I focus on the first step: getting out of bed. Then I drink some water and get dressed. After that, I go out the front door and sit in my car. Before I know it, I'm at the beach, swimming togs on, ready to get started. And when I've gone to the trouble of dragging my still-half-asleep body all the way there, the chances of me backing out are non-existent.

The difference that this one simple practice has made in my life is astounding. From my energy levels, to my outlook, to my general ability to cope with life's challenges - I feel dramatically better than I did just a month ago. When I start off my day right (by overcoming one small challenge), everything just goes more smoothly for me.

Morning swims suit me because I like being in the water (even if the prospect isn't always so enticing!), but maybe you're different. You might do better with a solo walk, a regular gym session or some sort of daily meditation habit. Whatever you choose, choose **something**. Creating a better life starts with the decision to do things differently. It doesn't have to be a big change - it just needs to be enough to change your perspective. And believe me, it gets easier. Push yourself to build the habit. Keep working until it's ingrained. You'll soon reap the benefits in the months and years to come.

Momentum can be an enemy as well as an ally, but it's the most powerful motivational tool you've got if you can turn it to your advantage. Use whatever "hacks" you need to trick your lazy human brain into action... and let the very same laziness keep you going once you've begun.

Lesson Three: When In Doubt, Choose Growth

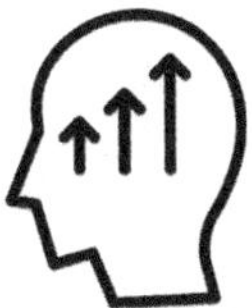

True courage isn't measured by how fearless a person is. It doesn't take courage to act on something you're not afraid of, after all. But being able to do something you *know* you're frightened of? That's courageous.

Life will test you in a lot of ways. Physically, emotionally, financially... different periods of life are marked by different sets of issues, and all take courage to overcome. But never let yourself feel guilty for the fear you experience.

When I was a young man, I thought of myself as a coward. Not because I was afraid of heights or girls or spiders, but because I feared other people learning who I really was. I hid behind a faux-masculine persona, a projection of what I thought other people wanted to see in me. And for years, I thought that meant there was something wrong with me. But there wasn't. Plenty of people felt the exact same as I did - like actors putting up fronts, following scripts that would make them seem likeable.

In learning to accept myself, I learned that feeling fear didn't make me a coward. In fact, it was the only thing that let me build my courage. Because in acting against that fear... in spite of how it told me to hide and run away... I discovered my true character.

We all face difficult decisions in life. No matter who you are or where you come from, it's guaranteed that life will present hurdles you'll never even have dreamt of. Having a solid set of guiding principles is one way to make scary choices seem more manageable; but if you need a mantra to cling to, let it be this one:

When in doubt, choose growth.

That doesn't mean to try things for the hell of it. If you're *doubting* someone's offer of cocaine, that's probably a sensible thing to do, and choosing to accept it when you don't want to is probably not the growth you're after. But if you're contemplating a change in scenery or life direction and the only reason you haven't tried it is that you're afraid of what it'll be like, that's probably a good sign that you should give it a go.

As individuals, we only grow when we press against the boundaries of what we *think* we're capable of. That's part of the reason why I got interested in self-improvement in the first place, actually. As a personal trainer and a once world-record holding powerlifter myself, the mental benefits I've gained (and inspired) from a simple gym routine have done wonders for my confidence. Bodybuilding and athletics are two of the simplest ways to expand your comfort zone - since they have tangible, physical ways to record progress (from mile times to personal-best lifts or muscle size), we can prove that our own limits are bullshit and expand our perception of what we think we're capable of.

As a kid, I never saw myself as one of *the* fit guys, and that remained true through secondary school as well. If you'd told me that I'd end up helping men to transform their bodies, I'd have laughed you off. But today, that's exactly where I am! By testing my limits in fitness, I learnt that those "limits" didn't really exist and I became more confident in every aspect of life as a result.

Growth doesn't always have to mean *"different"*, though. While it *is* only ever found outside your comfort zone and it probably is always going to scare you a little, it's not limited to new activities. If you're someone who does their best to blend in, it may very well be the case that refusing to change is your path to growth. This is the case for a lot of artists, for instance, who are told to abandon their dreams for a more sensible career path in adolescence. In that case, growth wouldn't come from kowtowing to teachers and parents, but from holding onto their dreams and ideals in the face of opposition.

The path to growth is different for everyone - pretty much the only constant is that, it'll always involve some internal struggle. So don't run from the things that frighten you. Find your fear, hug it tight... and move forward in spite of it.

Doing so is how you'll become truly courageous.

Lesson Four: Stop Hiding From Yourself

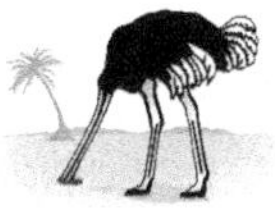

To give some context to this one, it's probably worth mentioning that I've struggled with addiction in the past... though probably not with what you're thinking.

I had a serious issue with internet pornography when I was a young man. But like any addict, I was in denial of my problem for a very long time. I rationalised it as a healthy coping mechanism, as something every man does when he's low and alone... but the truth is that I was just using porn to escape from my issues. Papering over the cracks in my self-image with cheap thrills and sexual fantasies I had no real interest in pursuing. And long after I kicked the habit, my past was still affecting me in many ways. My relationship with my wife suffered, as did my work.

Most addiction counsellors will tell you that heavy drinkers and drug users start abusing substances for similar reasons. Most are psychologically disturbed in one way or another, from issues like schizophrenia and undiagnosed BPD to things as mundane as depression or anxiety. To escape their pain, they turn to the quick hits of dopamine alcohol and narcotics provide. Most addicts know that this is a bad idea, but can't stop themselves from relapsing without outside help. It's the only way they know how to treat themselves.

But addictions only make mental problems worse. And that's not limited to substance abuse or porn addiction; most of us are addicted to something, if we're honest with ourselves. Whether that's social media, junk food, the 24/7 news cycle or external approval sought through lovers or friendships... nearly everyone's got something they can't let go of.

Nobody gets through life without collecting a few scars, and those scars make us vulnerable to developing unhealthy psyches. Most cope with their problems through seemingly benign addictions: through being a workaholic or a pathological bragger or an insatiable online shopper. But no matter how little physical "harm" an addiction causes, they're all equally bad for us. They're ways to hide from ourselves, and they're almost specifically designed to stop us from seeking help. It's like someone with chronic pain masking their symptoms with prescription painkillers to convince themselves they're healthy.

Ultimately, only you can determine the line between an addiction and a healthy form of stress relief. There are things people invest lots of time in (fitness, sports statistics, gaming, even sex) that don't automatically qualify as addictions. But if you look inside yourself and *know* that you're spending a lot of time on something because you can't stand the idea of what you are without it... well, it might be time to consider shelving the activity and seeking professional help.

Playing hide-and-seek with your issues is a losing game. The best way to "win" is to make sure you never play at all; but if you can't do that, the next best way is to confront your problems openly and truthfully and seek whatever help you need to resolve them. Don't shirk the work. No more Band-Aid solutions - focus on healing those wounds... or you'll suffer the consequences.

If this has resonated with you, I wish you the best of luck on your road to recovery. I've been where you are before, and I know how hard it is to get out. But you can and *will*, if you stay determined.

I believe in you.

Lesson Five: Learn From Your Struggles, But Don't Let Them Define You

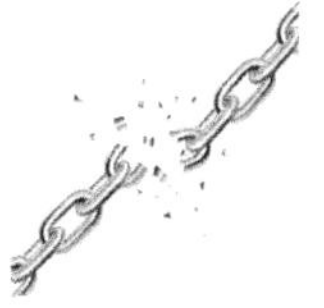

Everything in life is a learning experience. With the right mindset, you can draw immensely valuable knowledge from pretty much anything you go through. While the expression "what doesn't kill you makes you stronger" doesn't always apply in reality, there is some truth to the idea that we can learn a lot from seemingly negative experiences.

But it's very easy to start building a collection of emotional baggage alongside those lessons. And on some level, that might make sense. To spin a negative experience into an opportunity for growth, we've got to place some emotional significance on it and that usually means cementing or otherwise emphasising some of the pain we feel. In the quest for constant self-improvement, it's easy to draw important lessons from mistakes while also berating ourselves for them.

But you and I both know, that's not the path to wholeness. The past may have a lot to teach us, but that doesn't mean we should become mired in it.

Learn what you can from the things you've been through, accept the mistakes you've made... and move on. You'll make a lot more between now and the day you die, so you might as well get used to it.

Remember: it's human to make mistakes. You're not perfect. Neither am I. Neither is anyone! But if you're anything like me, you probably cut your friends and family a lot more slack than you give yourself... as if you're expecting yourself to be perfect, even when you know you're not. Lots of people do it. But like so many other bad emotional habits, excessive self-criticism being common doesn't make it *good* or *sensible.*

Use your experiences to make you better - not as another excuse to hurt yourself. You deserve more than that.

Lesson Six: Be As Happy As You Can Be

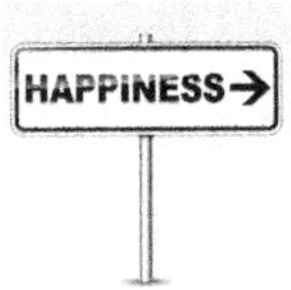

I've said it once, I've said it a thousand times - life's going to throw a lot of shit at you just for being you, and that's a fact we all need to accept. No matter who we are or how privileged our circumstances, we're all going to face our share of trials and tribulations. Some of them will seem unfair: they'll make us question the point of it all. They'll make us question ourselves. Others will seem like our own fault, even when they're not, and will make us hate ourselves a little more than society already encourages.

It's not easy being human. For as evolved and intelligent as our species is, there's a lot of debate over whether it's even possible for people to really *be* happy in the modern world. We're in a time of transition between the old and the new, and our whole species is struggling to find itself in a world torn between the natural and digital ages.

There's a reason that so many people today suffer from mental health issues, and it's not that the younger generations have *gone soft.* We're just becoming more aware of how difficult it is to find a sense of purpose that doesn't lend itself to destruction, like the spirits of nationalism and religious zealotry that defined the last 300 years.

But even so, it's our responsibility to carve out as happy an existence as we can for as long as we're alive. And contrary to popular philosophical belief, it's *not* impossible to be happy, no matter how chaotic the world becomes. Humans are an incredibly adaptable species - there's a reason we've risen to the heights we have.

But being happy isn't something that comes as a passive result of external success. That's why so many famous singers and film stars end up depressed, drug addicts or dead... they've chased the phantom of fame for so long because they think it'll make them happy, only to discover the opposite is true. Happiness isn't something you "get" like material wealth. It's something you build; something you earn through repeated good habits and mental framing.

This isn't a cure-all. Life is always bound to have some ups and downs; but if you're consistently experiencing downs, whether that's feeling depressed or not enjoying things like you used to, it's a sign that something needs to change. I'll always recommend professional help to anybody who's seriously worried about their mental health. Certain styles of therapy like CBT (cognitive-behavioural therapy) can do wonders for depression. But if you don't want to go that far, at least keep these tips with you as you go about your life.

1. **Never go to bed in the middle of an argument.** Anyone who's had a night-time argument with a partner will understand this one, but to keep it simple... sleeping when you're sad or angry is awful, and usually just makes a situation worse because your subconscious is given eight free hours to turn molehills into mountains while you sleep.

2. **Take care of yourself as if you were your own child.** Cook yourself healthy meals. Set a strict bedtime and *actually keep it.* Get yourself some exercise and fresh air every day. Audit who you're spending your time with and make sure they're

good for you. Our brain runs on biological processes; so make sure you're taking the best care of your body that you can.

3. **If you're an anxious type, both journalling and meditation are must-have habits.** The simplest way to engage with both is right before bed; carry out a "brain dump" of anything you're worried about a few minutes before you sleep, using pen-to-paper and follow it up with five minutes of quiet, uninterrupted focus on the breath. Give yourself permission to let your fears go while you meditate... and when you're done, hopefully you'll get enough off your chest via the brain-dump to get a good night's sleep.

Lesson Seven: Keep Your Eyes On The Stars...

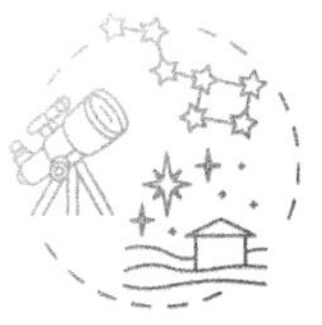

With how hard just being alive can feel sometimes, it's natural to feel some pessimism towards ourselves. But in the end, whether or not we choose to be hopeful is one of the only true choices we get in life.

No matter what life throws your way, you can get through anything as long as you have hope... and on the flipside, it's impossible to get through anything if you don't have it. The quality of hope defines us in more ways than we can ever understand, but learning how to harness its power is crucial in developing a healthy mindset.

In a way, learning how to be consistently hopeful is the ultimate goal of most people. It's not just about reaching personal satisfaction in the moment - we want to both be happy and believe that we'll continue to be, that it's more than a temporary high in a life filled with lows. We want assurance that the good things in life will last or that the bad things will fade. Honestly, finding fleeting moments of joy is easy even in the day-to-day grind. Sharing a joke with a friend, seeing cute dogs on the street, hearing children happy at play... these are all examples of moments that bring happiness to your day and doom-and-gloom a little easier to deal with.

But by themselves, moments like these aren't enough when viewed as isolated incidents. Viewing happiness as something to hunt or tune into puts too much pressure on ourselves to find it - happy moments turn to stressful ones as we wonder where we'll find the next. And for as long as we see happiness as a reprieve from 'reality', these moments of joy will actually make our lives *worse* than they would be without them.

Hope is the quality that'll save us from that fate. Learning to believe that these fleeting moments aren't hard to find and are actually just small manifestations of a constant, unending stream of goodness is what separates optimists from pessimists.

Joy is all around you. You just need to open your eyes and see.

It's not self-deception to believe that the world's a kind place. It's all a matter of perspective; how cruel or kind you perceive reality to be depends on what you call cruel or kind. And the world can seem like an awfully cruel place at times. War and famine... disease and hate... the 24/7 news cycle and the unending pain it pushes are just a few manifestations of our collective pessimism, but they're significant ones. It's hard to remember that life isn't just suffering when it's all we're presented with.

But the little moments of joy we find even in our darkest moments are all around us, always. There's always something good to be found in the world, in each other and in ourselves. All it takes is knowing where - and how - to look for it.

I can't tell you how to be happy or give you a step-by-step guide to anything as grand as infinite satisfaction. But I *can* tell you that the only way you'll get close to either is by learning to see the world through hopeful eyes again. Instead of trying to be Atlas and shouldering the burdens of the world, focus on bettering yourself and how you treat others. Know what you want out of life and *focus* on it. Remember that anything's within your reach when the right plan, timing, attitude meet a little perseverance, and that any limits you place on yourself are only as strong as your will to keep them there.

You're the master of your own destiny. You *choose* your future in everything you do, and happiness is just one choice of many.

You're not powerless to change how you feel.

Lesson Eight: But Watch Out For Potholes, Too

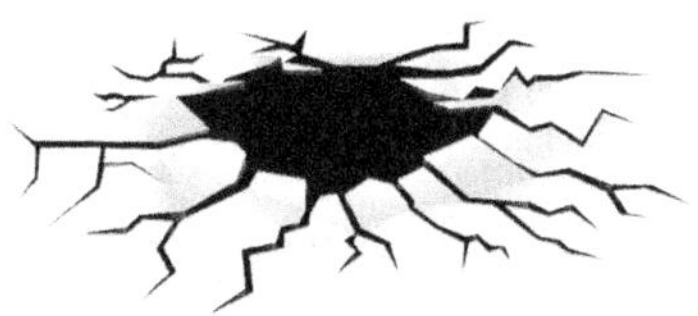

...But, that being said, *untempered optimism* is probably just as bad an idea as outright pessimism.

I stand by what I said in the previous section: I believe that life can be fundamentally kind for as long as we're prepared to view it as such, and the world can go from dreary to beautiful overnight if we learn to shift our requirements for beauty a little. But that attitude doesn't guarantee success or invincibility: optimism won't save you if you decide to walk in front of a fast-moving car, and hope won't get you through college if you never actually sit down to study.

Life, being what it is, loves to surprise the unprepared. And we're all unprepared, really, when we get down to it... but strict adherence to either hope or despair will ensure you're unprepared at a time when the opposite is most important. In a balanced individual, neither optimistic nor pessimistic (*read: hopeful or fearful*) thoughts completely dictate their actions.

Finding an equilibrium between the two is how sensible decisions are made - the famed middle ground of *realism,* which may as well be a no-man's land for how many of us embody it in our thoughts and behaviour. And with good reason. Realism is a hard mindset to adopt with the human brain's love of extremes - it's hard to work towards any goal without an accompanying chorus of "*this'll definitely work*" or "*this'll definitely fail.*" They're certainly catchier than "*This might work, if I create a solid plan and stick to it"* - but that doesn't make them right.

One of the most fantastically brutal things about life is that it's always exactly what we make of it. Whether you understand that as being a result of our physical actions or mental perceptions is irrelevant. Both schools of thought tell us that our locus of control is *internal* rather than *external*. This is why so many feel down on themselves. They take their poor living circumstances, emotional failures and career disappointments as proof of their worthlessness, since it's their own actions that have led them to that point... and some of you reading this may feel the same way. I did myself, as a younger man. I still do, sometimes (but I don't believe it anymore... which is the critical difference).

This perspective is only a problem if you view life as a one-way street. So what if you're in a shitty situation right now? Does that mean you always will be? If you put in the work, you'll probably be able to change things. Maybe you'll have to work two jobs for a while to get out of your shitty apartment, or maybe you'll have to put up with loneliness if you ditch your lying partner... but things *can* change if you make them and if you're willing to put in the effort. Life's not a zero-sum game of joy or sorrow, and success isn't guaranteed by good intentions alone. But it *is* possible to make things better, no matter how bad they get, and a sensible mind will always see that things don't have to stay the same forever.

So while you shoot for the moon, reach for the stars and indulge in a variety of other high-altitude metaphors for success, remember to watch out for what you're going to land on. Keep a steady eye on the horizon - the strong winds of life will knock you off course if you don't. But no matter what storm you find yourself in, there's always a way out if you know where to look. That doesn't mean you should pitch yourself out of a falling rocket with nothing but happy thoughts to keep you afloat; but it'd be just as useless to cry and huddle with your hands over your eyes. Instead, you need to find the parachute, open the hatch and *jump.* Trust that it won't break on you, that it'll bring you safely to land... and do what you can from there.

Keep your eyes on the stars all you like.

Just make sure you watch out for potholes.

Lesson Nine: Whatever You're Doing, Do It Properly

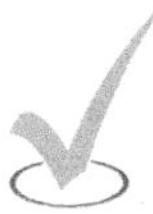

Before I found my calling as a men's coach, I worked a couple of different jobs: personal training, retail management, stay-at-home dad...

They weren't always easy. I certainly didn't wake up every morning raring to go, ready to give my A-game. I half-assed my duties a lot of the time and probably made life a lot harder for my colleagues (and kids) as a result. But as I grew more accustomed to working life and figured out how best to harness my motivation, I came to a realization:

Even if it's a task I don't care about, as long as I'm committed to it, I should always do it to the *best of my ability.*

To give a concrete reason why I think this is important, let's take a very physical example of shitty labour: cleaning public bathrooms.

I'm pretty sure bathroom cleaners don't love what they do. A lot of them are there for a paycheck and nothing more and to that end, the job is probably sufficient. But it's boring, unpleasant work, with minimal interaction and lots of physical labour if you're cleaning a big place. But would you bear those facts in mind if you walked into a public bathroom that looked like it hadn't been cleaned in months (as I'm sure many of us have)? Probably not. All you see is that the job isn't done and your day is all the worse for it.

Even when it feels like a job doesn't matter, it *will* to someone. When I worked in retail, I was often bored of dealing with employees and customers. The grind of re-stocking shelves every five minutes isn't a charming one. But I knew that any failure on my part to properly perform my duties would lead to a worse shopping and working experience for everyone who visited our shop... so I sucked it up and did my best until the day's end. If I expect people to do the same job for me when I need it, what gives *me* the right to half-ass it?

Whatever you're doing - in any sphere of life, be it a matter of fitness, career or romance - do it right. If you say you're going to do something, follow through and do it to the best of your ability. Even if your best changes on a daily basis (and sometimes, you'll feel like it does), all that matters is you *try* to respect the task and do as well as you can with what you're given.

That doesn't mean you should settle for menial labour or a rude partner - I'm not saying *"Someone has to do it, so why shouldn't it be you?"* But when you've agreed to do something, even if it's just a private promise... you owe it to *yourself* as much as anyone else to give it your best shot.

Lesson Ten: The Key Is In Your Pocket

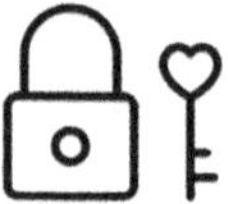

If life is a journey with death as its fixed destination, the only difference in peoples' lives is how they choose to get there. Some will walk a winding road, taking the time to smell the roses. Others will rush to the finish, taking fast cars and expensive trams to absorb as much of the fleeting scenery as possible.

Both travellers will reach the same place, eventually. But the routes they choose couldn't be any more different.

Ultimately, how you live your life is up to you. It's *your choice* how you want to spend the time you have in this world. But if you're not careful, that choice will be made for you. You'll be shuttled onto a path you've had no say in, and the only thing waiting for you at the end of *that* road is regret and anger. *Life is so unfair,* you'll rage. *Why did this have to happen to me? I was never given a choice in any of it.*

But the big secret to life that nobody wants to talk about is that choice isn't something *given* to you. It's something you just *have.*

No matter what life throws at you, your response to it is a choice you have to make. Whether you choose action or inaction, anger or sorrow or joy... they're all something you've chosen.

People will disagree with me on this one. They'll argue that because external events like redundancies, family bereavements and economic crashes can happen out of the blue. They'll say that life is inherently unpredictable and we have no control over it. And that may be true. As I write this (July 2020), we're in the midst of a global health pandemic. COVID-19 has disrupted our lives in ways we never could have predicted.

But our internal worlds are what colour our perception of reality and they *are* within our control. Ever thought about something/someone irritating from your past for so long that you start getting mad about them again? I sure have.

So even though emotions can arise unexpectedly (fear, pain and anger are all pretty quick-acting and reactive), our engagement with them is wilful in every circumstance. Even if it doesn't feel like it, time spent in meditation or engaging with stoic philosophies (the ones that aren't emotionally repressive) will help you to understand how thoughts and feelings don't define us. So even if the outside world is an unpredictable, uncontrollable place, your internal world doesn't have to be. You can travel the highways of life in what feels like a stuffy prison bus... or an emotionally intelligent Mercedes.

The driver's seat is yours. The key is in *your* pocket.

If you take nothing else away from this book, let that be the one thing you do.

Epilogue

We've come a long way together.

This book is a quick read. If I've included something here, it's because I believe it'll help you see real results as fast as possible. So, rather than attempting to summarise everything you've read so far, let me leave you with this final point:

On the road to self-acceptance, don't forget to forgive yourself.

While learning to overcome rejection-fuelled thoughts won't be easy, it'll be even harder if you don't forgive yourself for having them. Too often on the road to self-improvement, we learn to hate the person we used to be. We call the "old version" of ourselves worse, weak and inferior to spur ourselves forward. It's a natural instinct to look back on who we were ten, five or even *two* years ago and feel embarrassed about the mistakes we made...

but no matter how much you want it to, that shame won't propel you onwards. In fact, if you don't shed it, it'll just be more baggage holding you back.

I remember what it was like to be a cringey teenager. I remember what it was like to be a stupid(er) young(er) man. Sometimes, I find myself reacting angrily to memories of those times, and pile aggression onto the versions of me I'm desperate to forget. But guess what? While people can and do change, the past is set in stone. No amount of anger will erase the mistakes you're embarrassed by - and that's for the best. Those "mistakes" were actually a necessary part of your journey. Even if it doesn't feel like it, you would *not be* who you are now without making those mistakes. And if who you are now is perfectly, acceptably you... then so are your past mistakes.

Take accountability, sure. Learn not to make those mistakes again. But don't hate yourself for them, and don't hate what they've made you. Understanding how pointless that hatred is will make it easier to mend relationships damaged by pride or arrogance. Here's a personal example: after I graduated college, I found it hard to maintain relationships with the friends I made there. They reminded me of bad times; of the version of myself I didn't want to be... so I pushed them to one side. Since starting down this path of self-acceptance, I've reconnected with them. I've missed a lot, but we're finally making up for lost time.

And remember; there's always someone who'll love you in spite of and maybe *because* of, what your mistakes made you. Parents, partners, children, friends... take your pick.

The parts of yourself you reject for being "bad" may be the exact reason they love you so much. Who are you to say they're wrong for thinking it's okay?

The road ahead isn't an easy one. But it's a worthwhile one. In learning to deal with rejection properly, you'll set yourself up to become a better man - one who's capable of living the life of your dreams.

Put these ideas to work. Leave the baggage of the past in the past. Bust those old emotional ghosts. Don't be afraid to face who you are and what you've done. It's only by being honest with ourselves that we can grow.

A final quote to keep in mind:

"Do not go where the path may lead, go instead where there is no path and leave a trail".

Ralph Waldo Emerson

The path before you is not one that many have walked... but it's worth walking all the same. So begin your journey today and leave a trail for those who might follow. Friends, family, strangers - all stand to learn from your example.

All you need to do is take the first step, and let the process handle the rest.

Yours in strength,

Gavin

Next Steps

If you yould like to avail of additional supports going forward, I help men change their bodies, strengthen their minds and transform their lives.

There's a number of different ways I can help you achieve your goals. To find out more, check out Gavinmeenan.com and see how I can serve you best.

You can also get in touch with me via Instagram @gavinmeenan

About the Author

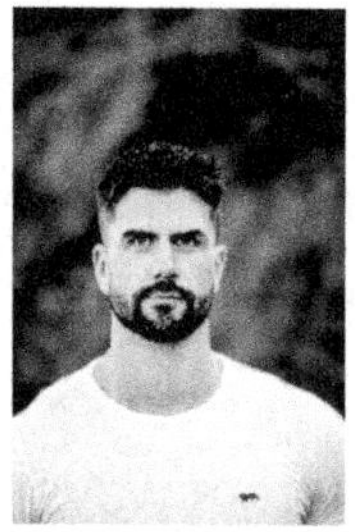

Gavin Meenan is an acclaimed personal transformation coach and founder of the Modern Warrior Academy. His work has reached a global audience of over 100,000 people.

During his early days as a personal trainer, Gavin learned that what sets us up for success is not just how well we move - it's how well we can manage our minds. That proved as true for his clients as it did for himself. The insights Gavin gained into peak performance psychology helped propel him to a European Powerlifting Championship win in 2016.

Through his struggles with addiction, depression and self-doubt, Gavin learned crucial lessons about what it means to accept yourself - and the dangers of self-rejection. He now passes those lessons on through his content on social media, podcasts, interviews, informative videos, books, workshops and more.

His first book, “Stronger Mind, Stronger Body, Stronger Life” was an Amazon Best Seller. Providing a holistic look at what it means to become stronger (hint: there’s more to it than lifting lots of weight in the gym), the book has helped men & women everywhere live better lives.

When he’s not working with clients, training or writing his next book, you’ll find Gavin enjoying the scenic surroundings of his West of Ireland home with his family.

Please Review

Dear Reader,

If you found this book helpful, would you kindly post a short review on Amazon or Goodreads? Your feedback will make all the difference to getting the word out about this book.

To leave a review, go to Amazon and type in the book title. When you have found it go to the book page, please scroll to the bottom of the page to where it says 'Write a Review' and then submit your review.

Thank you in advance.

Made in the USA
Las Vegas, NV
23 December 2021